Lydia Jane Roberts

Lydia Jane Roberts:

Nutrition Scientist, Educator, and Humanitarian

Margaret D. Doyle, Eva D. Wilson

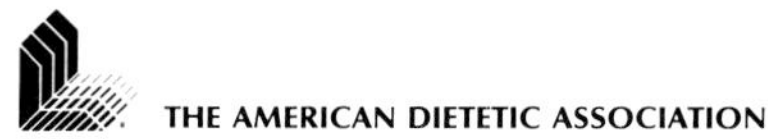

Library of Congress Cataloging-in-Publication Data

Doyle, Margaret D., 1914–
Lydia Jane Roberts / by Margaret D. Doyle, Eva D. Wilson.
p. xx, cm.
Includes bibliographical references.
ISBN 0-88091-047-X
1. Roberts, Lydia Jane. 2. Nutritionists—United States—Biography. I. Wilson, Eva D. II. Title.
TX350.8.R63D68 1989
613.2′092—dc20
[B] 89-17738
CIP

ISBN: 0-88091-047-X

CONTENTS

FOREWORD

In October 1924, I met Lydia Roberts in her office at the University of Chicago. I had just moved to the city and, almost before I was unpacked, I made an appointment to see her. Her early publications had intrigued me, a budding nutritionist, and I could hardly wait to make her acquaintance. Before we parted that day, I had registered for the course she called "Nutrition Work With Children." She spoke of other prospects that might interest me, and mentioned particularly that she needed library help with a book she was writing, which would carry the same name as her course. It was the beginning of a personal and professional association that lasted more than 40 years.

Friends who observed Lydia Roberts throughout her professional life were constantly amazed at her remarkable record of accomplishments. What made her such a dynamic force? What made her stand out from the crowd? I venture to suggest a few of the traits that appear to have shaped her approach to life. First, LJR had an innate ability to envision the future professional significance of current nutrition developments—activities and programs that would be common practice a half-century later. She was probably the first to recognize the importance of nutrition in the total health service spectrum. In effect, she anticipated today's multidisciplinary approach to nutrition education. She was indeed ahead of her time. LJR was not a visionary—far from it. She was a dreamer with a purpose. She had an incredible ability to communicate her ideas to people of all ages and backgrounds. She always knew exactly where she was going and what she expected to accomplish. This intellectual drive was basic to the tone of her leadership and her patterns of activity. In most cases her objective was the nutritional betterment of humanity, particularly of children.

Coexistent with her foresight was Lydia Roberts's indomitable spirit, which carried her beyond the goals most people set for themselves. *Determined, ener-*

getic, and *resourceful* were among the terms used by associates to characterize her spirit. Once she had decided to undertake a project, no amount of effort deterred her. Effort, in her case, meant doing anything that needed to be done. This biography is rich in accounts that exemplify her glorious spirit. Her efforts ran wide and deep, extending from the classroom to the research site; covering the counseling of educators, administrators, and heads of state; and including an endless range of nutrition programs around the world. To LJR, the lowliest tasks necessary to successful implementation were as important as the more exciting aspects of planning and organization. These were the directions in which Lydia Roberts's energies led her. This was her spirit in action.

Overshadowing all else in LJR was her personal magnetism, which contributed immeasurably to everything she did. She loved life. She had an eagerness to explore new ideas, a consuming interest in people and things, and a great capacity for friendship. People were important to her. She wanted them around her. Her vitality and zest for life were infectious. She imbued others with some of her own physical and mental vigor and drew people into her own areas of interest. She gave generously of herself, but she also expected and received much from associating professionally and personally with others. More than most people, LJR approached work and play with equal enthusiasm. Both were essential to her. Those around her came to share her outlook. Out of such relationships grew lifetime bonds of friendship that left permanent impressions on others and often affected their personal programs and professional careers.

We are indebted to the authors of this biography of Lydia J. Roberts. They have made LJR live again for all of us. Their own personal and professional experiences and those of classmates and associates have provided a compelling account of a long and productive career. They have reminded us, too, of the extent to which Dr. Roberts has spoken for herself. Few professional people have written so extensively or over so long a period as did LJR. Her writings constitute a considerable segment of nutrition history, and LJR was an important part of it. Her publications reflect her knowledge, her beliefs, her practices, and her dreams. It is impossible to separate Lydia Roberts, the person, from the events she helped to create. Together, they have influenced the thinking and the actions of the many people she touched throughout her long life. No one who was exposed to her teachings will forget or disregard them. Her teachings will be passed on through countless channels to future generations. This is LJR's legacy! Her biography has impressed us anew with Lydia J. Roberts as a remarkable human being who has left a lasting imprint on the world in which she lived.

Ethel Austin Martin
Chicago

PREFACE

If Lydia Roberts were alive today, she probably would be astonished at the idea of anyone wanting to know of her past accomplishments. "They want to write my biography? Imagine!" she would exclaim. Indeed, as many of her friends and associates have commented, Dr. Roberts's thoughts were of the present and the future, not of the past.

These friends and associates—and there are many—felt differently about preserving Lydia Roberts's memory, however. They kept saying, "Someone should write a book about Dr. Roberts." And so, finally, we undertook the task.

Lydia Roberts was our professor, our adviser, our friend. Our admiration for her was great; we thought we knew her well. But, as we set about gathering information, we discovered a person greater than even we had realized. She was a person of many facets, of many accomplishments, but with one overriding goal that influenced all she did: to use her knowledge and skills, as she often said, "for human betterment." Her success is apparent, we think, in the pages of this book.

Since Lydia Roberts was oriented so much more toward the future than the past, it is not surprising that information on her early life is not readily available. Contemporaries who might have told about that life are no longer living. Even family members who remember her with great affection have little information about her. Early letters and photographs apparently were not saved. When she attended family get-togethers there seems to have been little discussion of her life in Chicago or in Puerto Rico. She was more concerned with the day-to-day activities of her nieces and nephews. A niece by marriage wrote that as she looked back on "Aunt Lyd's" visits, "it is her humility that impresses me the most—to the point where the family possibly didn't realize the scope of her work."

Fortunately, more information is available concerning Dr. Roberts's professional life from the time of her University of Chicago appointment onward. Many of her former students are still professionally active or are in early retirement. Many of the people who worked with her in Puerto Rico were very young at the time, so their recollections are vivid.

Many people have helped provide information for this biography. A request for recollections about Dr. Roberts was made in the form of a note in professional journals and a letter to all University of Chicago alumni for whom addresses were available. Responses came from more than 50 former students and professional associates in the United States. In Puerto Rico, Dr. Roberts's friends were generous with both their time and their help in many ways: recounting their experiences, making the files in the Sala Roberts available, arranging a trip to Doña Elena.

Although Lydia Roberts apparently was not a letter saver herself, some of her friends were. A series of letters from Dr. Roberts to her close friend, Ethel Austin Martin, covers the entire time she was in Puerto Rico. These letters, written in Dr. Roberts's lively style, have been particularly helpful not only in giving an account of the work of those years, but in providing insight about Lydia Roberts as a person. Another illuminating series of letters was written by Dr. Roberts to Ramonita Ramos, her secretary at the University of Puerto Rico. These letters were intended for the whole Department of Home Economics faculty. They usually contained some items of business, but were also delightful, newsy accounts of her trips away from Puerto Rico. Unless noted otherwise, all of the quotes from Dr. Roberts come from these two collections of letters. A collection of letters and reports furnished by Thelma Dreis was very helpful, as were the reports on the activities of the Puerto Rico Nutrition Committee provided by Dr. Esther Seijo de Zayas. Dr. Audrey Maretzki turned over for our use an unpublished manuscript, "Where Every Prospect Pleases," which proved very useful, since it contained material from some of Dr. Roberts's files that are no longer available. Other sources of information have included material obtained from interviews, from the archives of the University of Chicago, and from the Medical Center Library of Vanderbilt University.

Many of the letters from and conversations with students and friends have been quoted in this biography. Although the source of each quotation has not been identified individually, the people who contributed are included below.

All the following people—family, former students, university faculty, professional associates, friends, and admirers of Lydia Roberts—contributed through letters, conversation, research, or editorial assistance to the making of this book. We offer our sincere thanks to all of them.

Lena Bailey; Marie Balsley; Esther Batchelder; Anita Barr; Wilma Beckman Belser; Barbara Bowman; Eva Boggs Callaghan; Margaret Chaney; Miriam

M. Chavez; Faith Clark; Marta Coll de Velázquez; Lillian Colón de Reguero; William J. Darby, MD; Thelma A. Dreis; Jane Ebbs; Ruth White Engler; Annette Young Feldman; Katherine H. Fisher; Margaret S. Follstad; Marjorie Greider Foreman; Olive McKay Fraser; Elsa Haglund; Esther Thornton Taylor Hall; Margaret Harrington; Catherine Hastie; Ruth L. Huenemann; Ann Goodhue Hunt; Virginia Jauch; Margaret Maxwell Kleiber; Graham B. Ladd, MD; Ruth M. Leverton; Mary Lewis; Ethel Locke; Rayna DeCosta Loewy; Miriam E. Lowenberg; Louise Majonnier; Margaret W. Mangel; Audrey Maretzki; Ethel Austin Martin; Milla Newland; Isabel T. Noble; Jessie Obert; C. D. O'Connell; Hazel O'Connor; Helen G. Oldham; Celéste H. Perez; Ruth L. Pike; Margarita Pont Flores; Ramonita Ramos; Elouise Smith Rice; Katherine P. Riddle; Jean A. S. Ritchie; Marguerite Robinson; Una Lane Robinson; Sylvia Rodríguez de Santiago; Mary Marguerite Rooney; Bernice Hopper Roth; Elizabeth Sánchez; Carmen Luz Santiago de Ramos; W. H. Sebrell, MD; Esther Seijo de Zayas; M. Ella Siddell; Alice McLean Jones Stewart; Julia M. Tandy; E. Neige Todhunter; Mable Pashley Tompkins; Rosa Marina Torres; Nívea Torres-Naficy; Ruth Tucker; Lizette Vincens de Sánchez; Margaret Hodo Walburn; Ruth Jones Wilson; Robert Wissler, MD; Mertie Cook Wolverton; Bernice Wait Wood; Elizabeth Burrus Woodard.

Acknowledgment also must be made for the help of those who read, criticized, and supplemented the first version of the manuscript: Dr. Neige Todhunter, Dr. Helen Oldham, Dr. Ruth Pike, Dr. Katherine Fisher, Dr. Miriam Lowenberg, Mrs. Lillian Colón de Reguero, Dr. Esther Seijo de Zayas, and C. D. O'Connell.

Finally, we offer very special thanks to Mrs. Ethel Austin Martin, whose enthusiastic help and cooperation have been with us at every stage of the preparation of the biography. Without her encouragement, it is doubtful that the task would have been accomplished! It has been a privilege to work with her.

Margaret D. Doyle
Eva D. Wilson

PROLOGUE

Lydia Jane Roberts was born 30 June 1879 in Barry County, Michigan. When she was a small child, her family moved to Martin, in Allegan County, about 50 miles north of Kalamazoo. She graduated from Martin High School in 1898. She attended normal school in Mount Pleasant, Michigan, where she received a teaching certificate in 1899. She taught in rural schools in Michigan for several years.

Up to this point, the biography of Lydia Roberts would be little different from that of many other bright young women of the period. Women were attending college in increasing numbers, and an increasing number were also achieving some working experience, frequently as teachers. Even so, the norm for most women still was to marry and settle down, often in the towns where they grew up.

But Lydia Roberts was different. Although she always remembered her life in Michigan with pleasure and nostalgia, settling down in Martin was not enough for her. She left Michigan for Montana, where she taught in Great Falls and in Miles City. She returned to Michigan for a second, more advanced, teaching certificate, and, in 1910, went back to Montana. She taught third grade in Dillon and also served as critic teacher in the normal school there (now Western Montana State College). To have settled down in this interesting and challenging job would have been satisfying for many women.

But Lydia Roberts was different. A practical, down-to-earth kind of person, she was concerned not only for the education of her pupils, but also for their health and welfare. It was her opinion, based on a variety of observations, that not all of the children she saw in the course of her work were as strong and healthy as they should be. She became convinced that part of the problem, at least, was due to their food habits. This was an era when many school children—farm children, particularly—missed the main family meal, the noontime dinner. "Lard-pail" lunches and cold suppers probably were often insufficient to meet their needs. Possibly other teachers had made similar observations, but had felt that little could be done to change the situation.

But Lydia Roberts was different. Perhaps she had read of some of the discoveries in the new science of nutrition. Perhaps she felt that change was possible, but realized that before she could be effective in bringing about such change she needed to know more about child health and children's food needs. In 1915, at age 36, she left Montana to return to the Middle West and to enroll in the Department of Home Economics in the College of Education at the University of Chicago. Two years later she received a baccalaureate, and, after another year, the degree of Master of Science. She became a member of the faculty of the University of Chicago, continuing her studies while on the job. In 1928, when she was 49, she received the degree of Doctor of Philosophy. In 1930 she became head of the Department of Home Economics and Household Administration at the university. She had a distinguished career in teaching, in research, and in public service, remaining at the University of Chicago until 1944, when she reached the mandatory retirement age of 65. For most people this would be the climax of professional life. Retirement would bring a change in lifestyle, the chance to do volunteer work, or just to get some well-deserved rest after a satisfying career.

But Lydia Roberts was different. During a brief wartime assignment in Puerto Rico (at the request of M. L. Wilson of the National Nutrition Committee), she had made a great impression on island officials. Early in 1944, Chancellor Jaime Benítez of the University of Puerto Rico asked her to join the staff of the university. After some consideration, she agreed to go for a six-month period, starting after her retirement in June. But six months were not nearly enough time—she never left. In 1946 she became professor and chairman of the Department of Home Economics, a position she held until 1952, when she retired once again. Even in her second retirement she remained active, however, teaching at the university, taking part in Caribbean workshops and in international seminars, acting as a consultant for the Food and Agriculture Organization, working on a nutrition textbook for students in the Caribbean area, and, most important, initiating the Doña Elena project, a demonstration in community development that became a model for many projects in other parts of the world. On 28 May 1965, while working in her office at the University of Puerto Rico, she collapsed. She died within a few hours, without ever having the feeling of being "on the shelf." Her third career was finished. The body of the small-town girl from Michigan was returned home for burial in the family plot in Martin.

Yes, Lydia Roberts *was* different. Few people have had as much influence on the practical, applied side of nutrition education and research as this three-career woman. This difference is the reason why Dr. Roberts's former students, professional associates, and many friends want to join together in preserving her memory in this biography.

CHAPTER 1

Lydia Roberts, the Person

Martin, Michigan, is a pleasant small town set in the rolling farmland of southern Michigan, just about halfway between Kalamazoo and Grand Rapids. According to people who live there, Martin has not changed much over the years. Garages and filling stations, of course, have replaced livery stables and blacksmith shops. Storefronts have been modernized. The trees that arch over the streets are bigger. There are new school buildings, and one of the early residences, the big house on the corner of Tenth and Lee streets, has been converted into a popular restaurant.

Two main streets, Tenth and Allegan, intersect to form the business district. Within a couple of blocks of this intersection, business gives way to homes—simple, substantial, sturdy. Many of the houses, especially those nearest the main intersection, were built in the early days of the town, and many of the families who live in Martin today are descendents of the Scottish Presbyterians who founded the town around 1836.

It was in one of the big white houses on Allegan Street that Lydia Jane Roberts grew up. She was a small child when her parents moved from Hope Township in Barry County, where Lydia had been born on 30 June 1879. She had two older sisters, Mary ("Mame") and Lillian ("Lil"). The youngest child, John, was born after the family had moved to Martin. Warren Roberts, her father, was a carpenter who helped to build many of the houses in Martin. Mary Jane Roberts, her mother, like most women of her time, kept the house and took care of the children.

Lydia Roberts's childhood years probably were typical of those of many girls growing up in American small towns in the late 19th century. School, homework, and chores took up a lot of the time in winter, but no doubt there was time for such Michigan delights as sliding on snow-covered hills and ice skating. In the summer there was more time for fun, but still lots to be done—helping with the garden, with canning and preserving, with sewing clothes for the coming year.

One joy of Michigan summers, the wonderful fruit, was a cherished memory all her life. Many years later, when she had lived in Puerto Rico for some time, she wrote that she had really had to learn to like tropical fruits. Papayas and pineapple she liked "fairly well," she said, "but I'd give up all of them for strawberries, cantaloupe, blueberries and green apple sauce!"

Although there seem to be few family letters or photographs to document Lydia Roberts's childhood, one can imagine what she was like in those growing-up years. She was, perhaps, not pretty in the traditional sense of that time, but her face was undoubtedly animated by her interest in the people and the world around her. It is likely that she was a leader among her friends and at school, foretelling her outstanding leadership abilities of later years. Altogether, it probably was a very happy childhood. Certainly Lydia Roberts always remembered Martin with great affection.

As in all families, there were changes in the Roberts family over the years. Warren Roberts died in 1906 at the age of 55. In what must have been a great tragedy for the family, John, the only son, died just four years later, when he was only 24. Apparently he was the victim of some sort of accident. Mame married and left Martin to raise her family in Hastings. Lydia left home, first to go to normal school and later to work. Lillian, closest to Lydia in age, followed Lydia first to Montana and then to Chicago. Their mother, Mary Jane Roberts, was left alone in the big white house on Allegan Street. Actually, she was not alone much of the time, for she used to provide lodging for high-school girls from the country who arranged to stay in town during the worst months of the winter. Later, when Mame also was a widow, she came home to stay for a while, and Lydia and Lillian were frequent visitors from Chicago. After their mother's death in 1933, Lydia and Lillian kept the house for some time, staying there when they went home to Martin.

When Lydia and Lillian lived in Chicago, they traveled to Michigan frequently and often visited Mame and her family in the Hastings area. Mame had three children, whose growing up was watched with pleasure by their aunts. All three of Mame's children married and raised their own families in Hastings or nearby, and kept in close contact with their Aunt Lyd and Aunt Lil. Later, when Lydia came back to Chicago from Puerto Rico, she and Lillian always made a visit to the Michigan family. The joy Lydia felt in those visits was expressed in her letters to Puerto Rico:

> *I spent last week in Michigan, and saw all my family: Jack and Clementine and my sister Mame who lives with them; Mary Jane and Anne and their father and mother; my grand niece Anne and her three children, aged 3, 2 and 2 months; my grand nephew Tom and his four year old son, Pat*

(the cutest thing you ever saw); then, up in Greenville, my nephew Robert and his wife Hazel and [their] girls. . . drove to my old home town of Martin and saw my few remaining friends there, then to Grand Rapids. . . pretty good for a week!

Despite Lydia's full schedule, she seems to have found time on some trips for other activities. "Sunday Jack and I went nutting," she wrote in an October letter. "He took the old truck and drove to the back lot. We gathered over three bushels of hickory nuts and one of butter nuts. Nutting was always one of my favorite fall occupations and it seemed quite like old times."

One of her letters to Puerto Rican friends closed with the comment, "I don't know why I think you'd be interested in my family visits—except to know I saw them all and had a good time." But the Puerto Ricans loved hearing about the visits, because they knew how important family ties were to their friend.

When they were living in Chicago and made trips back to Martin, Lydia and Lillian usually took some of their Chicago friends with them. Often the visits would include some typical Michigan activity such as going to an orchard to pick apples, and would be followed by a picnic or supper arranged by friends in Martin—childhood playmates who remained lifelong friends. The "Roberts girls" (as they are still referred to in Martin) enjoyed having their two worlds meet.

It is certain that Martin and the house on Allegan Street always meant a great deal to Lydia Roberts. It also seems certain that many of the characteristics that friends and students associated with her—her prodigious capacity for work, her thrift, her sense of humor, her liking for people—all were influenced by the years spent in Martin.

Lydia and Lillian, the two middle children in the Roberts family, had a close association throughout their lives. For many years they shared an apartment on Blackstone Avenue in Chicago, just a short distance from Lydia's office in Emmons Blaine Hall at the University of Chicago, and a short walk to the Illinois Central station where Lillian took the train to the loop office where she was a secretary.

Many former students recall with pleasure the times they were invited to the Robertses' apartment for a meal or for a department party. Students who were a long way from home often were favored by an invitation to Thanksgiving dinner—a traditional meal with all the trimmings, undoubtedly reminiscent of holiday dinners in the family home in Martin. The sight of the usually dignified, well-groomed, well-dressed Dr. Roberts bustling about the kitchen, her dress covered with a big apron, stirring the gravy or mashing the potatoes, beaming over the perfectly cooked turkey, was reassuring to those who up until that time had regarded her not only with respect, but with considerable awe.

Even more to be desired was an invitation to spend a day at the cottage in the Indiana Dunes on the southern tip of Lake Michigan, about 45 miles from Chicago. Lydia Roberts and another faculty member, Evelyn Halliday, owned the cottage jointly, having bought it in 1928 from Katharine Blunt, the former head of the Home Economics Department at the University of Chicago. Dr. Roberts loved to share the beauty and the outdoor activities of the ever-changing dunes and lake. "Frequently, on balmy Friday afternoons," a colleague wrote, "she would gather together four or five companions and take off for the cottage in the dunes."

For Lydia Roberts, the cottage was not only a place for recreation, but also a quiet retreat for work, and that aspect was also shared with others. When one student was working on her doctoral dissertation and trying at the same time to incorporate the data into an article for publication, Dr. Roberts invited her to come out to the cottage to work. "She had her special work to do, too, but helped me evaluate the results as they evolved," the student wrote. "It was a fun week as well as a working week. . .we also spent time in relaxing and chatting, talking of many things."

Sharing the Blackstone Avenue apartment with her sister was an especially fortuitous arrangement for the always-busy Lydia, for apparently Lillian took over much of the responsibility for running the household. A letter from a former student commented, "Dr. Roberts received much help from her sister. . . . I remember someone saying that the sister packed her bags, and did other things for her which a wife usually does for a husband, hence Dr. Roberts could accomplish much more in her profession." Student rumor also had it that Lillian picked out Lydia's clothes, becomingly simple suits and dresses, often in a soft shade of blue that set off her blue eyes and, later on, her silver-gray hair. After her move to Puerto Rico, Lydia Roberts changed her style. She cut her hair, got a permanent, and often wore dresses of brighter colors. Perhaps this was just a commonsense reaction to the tropical climate, or perhaps she was expressing her own tastes in a more lively manner. Lillian never moved to Puerto Rico, although she made long visits there. The sisters remained very close, however, and Lillian often still shopped for Lydia in Chicago.

After she went to Puerto Rico, Lydia undoubtedly missed the kind of day-to-day help she was used to having from Lillian. Competent as she was as a professional, she seemed to be somewhat at a loss in setting up her daily life in the new setting. When she first went to the island, she really had not committed herself to staying permanently, and she had a variety of temporary living arrangements. It was not until 1949 that she moved into the hotel apartment in Santurce that was to be her home for many years.

In letters from Puerto Rico to a Chicago friend, Dr. Roberts frequently commented on the cost of everyday items and on the time required for shopping. In 1946 she wrote, "You've no idea how hard it is to assemble just essentials. There's no such thing as just going to Fields and ordering the whole lot sent out. It has to be a personal search for each item to locate the store that has it in San Juan, Santurce or Rio Piedras."

It's not surprising that shopping in Puerto Rico in the immediate postwar years was more difficult than in Chicago. Even later on, however, she seemed to retain some of the same feelings, and was often shocked at the prices—apartment rents, for example. Apparently Lillian was still consulted on these matters, for on more than one occasion, when considering some expense, Lydia would say, "'but what's money for,' Lil always asks me."

These ideas of thrift, doubtless instilled in her youth in Martin, stood Dr. Roberts in good stead in running a university department and in getting the most out of every dollar in a research grant. Thriftiness was invaluable in Puerto Rico. She could understand the attitudes of people with limited funds and she was full of practical ways to help make money go further. The story is told of how, on seeing a pile of discarded cans outside a school-lunch kitchen in Puerto Rico, she started asking everyone she met, "What can be made with old cans?" Many imaginative, useful and practical suggestions were made—measuring equipment, stovepipes, cups, plates, water containers. As a result:

> *. . . a group of industrial arts teachers was summoned to a Saturday morning workshop sponsored by the Home Economics Department of the University of Puerto Rico. With virtually no outlay of funds the school lunchroom trash heaps were transformed into gold mines of useful items for homes where money could buy only the barest essentials.*[1]

Lydia Roberts always remained cost-conscious. It was just one of her little idiosyncracies, like refusing to tell her age. Apparently, when she was asked to fill out any form that requested age, she would simply write "adult" or "over 25"—that was enough, she said. Sometimes there were problems. In 1955, she went as a Food and Agriculture Organization consultant to Uganda. She filled out all the necessary forms, except, of course, for her age. FAO staff members who knew Dr. Roberts and who were anxious to have her go to Uganda knew there was no use asking her for the information. The medical officer, on the other hand, could not understand why her age was not included. He approved her appointment, finally, indicating that she seemed suitable for the job "whatever her age may be." He might have been surprised, had he known he had approved the appointment of a 76-year-old woman! But then, this woman wrote of herself, when she was 81, "the odd part is that I don't *feel* I belong in the *old* group (except when I look in the mirror!)"

Associates of Dr. Roberts were impressed with her capacity for productive work. Indeed, it was common student speculation that, in order to accomplish so much, she must never sleep—or that there were more hours in her days than in those of ordinary mortals. Obviously, saving time was just as important to Lydia Roberts as saving money. She did not waste time, but used it efficiently, just as she did every dollar. If she had a few spare minutes—in an airport, for example, or waiting for an appointment, or for someone to pick her up to go out for dinner—she always filled the time. She wrote letters, she made notes for future reports, she planned her next activities. She was a believer in "getting at things" and "keeping at" jobs until they were finished. She moved briskly. She was an early riser who usually arrived at her office well before 8:00 AM, which she considered the official start of her day. "Dr. Roberts did not require much time for sleep," one of her Puerto Rican associates said. She went on to recount how after one long, tiring day in the field, Dr. Roberts's young coworkers all came to work a little later than usual the next morning, because they were sure Dr. Roberts would be tired and would not put in her customary early appearance. "It was a surprise," the associate said, "to find her already at work at her desk when they arrived."

Toward the end of her life Dr. Roberts did complain sometimes of "being slow"—sounding sad, and a little surprised. It would appear, however, that none of her younger colleagues ever spent much time waiting for her! Occasionally, in her letters, there were indications that she felt she had too much to do. But she could deal with that with humor. One student wrote of how Dr. Roberts had once told her, "There are so many people wanting me to do so many things, sometimes I feel like I'm being chased by a pack of dogs—but, I just carry along a few bones, and every now and then I throw one to the nearest dog."

One reason for her tremendous capacity for work was that she really enjoyed what she was doing. It was interesting and worthwhile, which gave her a feeling of satisfaction. However, life was never "all work and no play" for her. She could put her work aside for other things she enjoyed with equal gusto. She loved the theater, good movies, mystery stories, Scrabble games, favorite radio programs, good food, good conversation—and good friends with whom to share them.

Lydia Roberts had a tremendous capacity for making and keeping friends, both personally and professionally. Things she enjoyed—trips to the dunes, to Martin, or, later, beautiful drives in Puerto Rico—were all better when shared with others. She was a tireless letter writer, with a gift for making what she wrote about come alive. She loved receiving letters, too, though her friends did not always do as well as she when it came to writing. In one of her letters to Puerto Rico she said, "It's nice having friends who'll do things for you—even if they don't write!" On her trips to the States her days seemed to be filled with luncheon and dinner engagements—one thing she always enjoyed was meeting friends for lunch at Marshall Field's department store. She usually tried to arrange her visits so that she could attend meetings of the American Institute of Nutrition in the spring, or meetings of The American Dietetic Association in the fall. The meetings were interesting, of course, but her greatest pleasure was in seeing her friends. After one meeting of The American Dietetic Association she wrote, "I've got a list of about a hundred former students and friends that I saw."

Just occasionally—not often—something Dr. Roberts did for fun prevented her from making her usual careful preparations for class. One student wrote:

> *One day she entertained us with an account of her visit to the Chinese Opera. If I remember correctly, she attended it in Chinatown with ChiChe Wang. We were sure she had not had time to prepare a formal lesson that day, and were enchanted with her account of the actors, their running up and down, their singing, costumes, etc Although that was a day when we learned little nutrition, we learned a lot of Lydia J. Roberts and loved her for it.*

More often, students and coworkers were impressed (and sometimes a little chagrined) by the amount of preparation she made for classes, meetings, or conferences. Dr. Franklin Bing, in his memorial essay on Lydia Roberts published in the *Journal of Nutrition* in 1967, had this to say concerning a meeting of a committee dealing with child nutrition for the 1929 White House Conference on Children:

> *Her subject was the caloric requirements of children. She passed around some mimeographed sheets which contained a great mass of information having to do with everything that had ever been written on the subject. I was impressed, and I think others were also impressed, especially some of the clinicians whose presentations had been casually sketchy. . . . I remember on the train ride back. . . Dr. Shohl's telling me of the excellent work being done by the Chicago women. He did not need to tell me that the Roberts' report on calories had stimulated at least one member of the Committee to put extra effort into his own assignments.*[2]

The upbeat, enthusiastic side of Lydia Roberts's nature was the one most familiar to her friends and associates. Many of them might have been surprised to know that she sometimes felt lonely and out of things. In her early years in Puerto Rico, an atmosphere greatly different from the culture to which she was accustomed, she sometimes wrote of the dullness of her life, her lack of companionship there, and the discouragement she sometimes felt. In 1946 she wrote, "I do nothing but work 8–5, supper, drive along the ocean or see a movie, read a mystery, go to bed and repeat the next day. So you see it's not very exciting."

A short time later she wrote, poignantly, "I must close this and drive to the Post Office and mail it and a letter to Lil. That is a regular Sunday evening performance—but tonight, I go alone, and it's dark!" As time passed, her loneliness lessened, but it was still there sometimes. On 24 December 1956 she wrote of her plans for Christmas, "So far as I know I shall have a full day when I feel free to read and loaf, with no conscience reminding me I should work." Her lack of Christmas plans was perhaps not as depressing to her as it might have been, for she had remarked in previous years that "it's terribly hard to make it seem like Christmas in the tropics."

Lydia Roberts may have had, as anyone does, her low moods, but probably they were fleeting. She was never a person to feel sorry for herself—her sense of humor helped her in that. No associate of Dr. Roberts can reminisce about her for very long without recalling that sense of humor. For former students, this side of her personality was one of their most cherished and most frequently mentioned memories. "She liked a good joke," one person wrote, "she liked a little sauciness, too." And, as some of the students commented in their letters, if the good joke was on her, that made it all the better for Lydia Roberts.

"She knew a lot of jingles," a former associate recalled, "and she would relate them at the drop of a hat, with a low chuckle . . . not in class, but supposing you were riding downtown to see someone for a business meeting or something like that, she kept you interested . . . .One I remember best of all was this:

"Bread and meat are good to eat,
Potatoes are not bad
But bread and milk's the food for me
It's good for any lad.
The old red cow, she gives the milk,
And mama bakes the bread.
I put the bread into my milk
And then into my head."

This young lad and his dietary habits form a recollection that perhaps goes back to her Martin days.

The jingles were remembered—indeed, quoted—by other students, as were anecdotes of her childhood, stories she used in class to illustrate points, or stories in which she laughed at herself. One story she told of her childhood was of how her mother had sent her to the store to get some pickles. In those days, pickles were kept in small barrels, covered with pickling brine. When the grocer asked if she wanted some of the liquor on the pickles, her answer was a firm no—because she had signed a pledge in Sunday School never to touch liquor!

It was not just the stories she told, however, but the way she told them that delighted her listeners. As Dr. Bing commented, "Her sense of humor, always evident, helped put others at their ease. . . . It was a feminine type of humor, reminding one of a little girl, watching the antics of the little boys out of the corners of her eyes, quietly chuckling, and then sharing her amusement with her friends afterwards."[2] The same style came through in her letters, many of which contained humorous descriptions, observations or anecdotes. There was, for instance, this comment on the name of one of her associates in Puerto Rico:

I mentioned Dr. Plough. How would you pronounce it?
In English, ough *may be:*
ow *as in plough*
o *as in dough*
uff *as in rough*
off *as in cough*
oo *as in through*
So he could be
Plow
Plo
Pluff
Ploff or
Ploo.
He is called all of them. I finally learned the correct one is Ploo.
Ain't the English language wonderful?

In her contacts with others—except for family and close friends—Dr. Roberts was usually briskly professional. However, her sense of humor served her well in these relationships also, for it revealed the warm, human side of her nature. It was not unusual for students, in their initial contacts with her, to see her as austere and self-contained rather than warm and outgoing. But for most, this feeling was soon dispelled by her genuine concern for and interest in them and their problems or successes. Whether it was finding a job or a fellowship for a needy student, an invitation to dinner for a lonely one, or words of encouragement for a disconsolate one, she seemed aware of them as individuals. "Only the people she helped can know how much she really did," one person said. They could respond, however, by doing their best. As one associate wrote, ". . . by her very being she demanded respect. Your duty was to do your very best so that you and Dr. Roberts shared a pride in your work."[1]

During the years when Dr. Roberts was at the University of Chicago, all of her graduate students were women. Men doing nutrition research at that time were generally in medicine or biochemistry, fields that were not then as open to women as they came to be later. During the 1920s and 1930s, an increasing number of women were taking graduate work and were seeking careers. Combining a career with marriage, although certainly not unheard of, was not as common as in later years. Unmarried herself, Dr. Roberts appeared to assume that students who married would automatically drop their career plans. A number of students wrote of feeling her "disappointment" when they married. For the marriage, her wishes were for happiness and success; the disappointment was for the missed career. As the years passed, many of the lost careers turned out not to have been lost at all. The growing number of students who successfully combined marriage, motherhood, and career must have been a source of satisfaction to her.

In her professional contacts with men, Dr. Roberts always got on well. The men admired her competence—but they, too, were sometimes a little in awe of her. One colleague told of how on one committee the distinguished male scientists who were Dr. Roberts's fellow committee members were all on a first-name basis with each other—but they were not quite sure how to address her. "The men couldn't quite see themselves calling Miss Roberts 'Lydia,' and yet they didn't want to call her the more formal title of Dr. Roberts or Miss Roberts. Finally they decided to call her 'Dr. Lydia,' and that's what she remained to those important men." The new title was taken up by some of her other associates, as well, for it seemed to solve a problem in an era where formality was giving way to greater ease in professional relationships. It probably pleased Dr. Roberts. "Dr. Lydia" no doubt seemed more friendly.

During the course of her professional life, Lydia Roberts received many honors and awards. Academically, these ranged all the way from undergraduate and graduate honor societies (Phi Beta Kappa and Sigma Xi) to the degree of Doctor of Laws conferred in 1958 by The Ohio State University. Her research in child nutrition was recognized by the Borden Award in 1938. Her work in the profession of dietetics brought her the Marjorie Hulsizer Copher Award, the highest honor of The American Dietetic Association, in 1952. The American Dietetic Association also named an annual essay contest in her honor. A compilation of these essays was published by the Association in 1968.[3] As a home economist, she was elected an honorary member of Omicron Nu in 1952. She was elected a Fellow of the American Institute of Nutrition in 1962. Her civic activities were recognized by the University of Chicago Alumni Association's Public Service Citation in 1945, and she was twice honored by the Altrusa Club in San Juan for her work in establishing home economics in Latin America. She was elected to the Chicago Senior Citizen's Hall of Fame in 1965. Her practical accomplishments in the field of child welfare were recognized in 1957 by the Marshall Field Award, which acknowledged her role in improving the nutrition of children in Puerto Rico. The award that may have been the most meaningful to her also came in 1957, when the government of Puerto Rico recognized her contributions to the improvement of public health and nutrition on the island by naming her Exemplary Citizen of the Commonwealth, its highest honor. This award had been given only once previously. She received it, together with the Marshall Field Award, in a ceremony at La Fortaleza, the governor's palace, from the hands of her good friend and staunch supporter, Luis Muñoz Marín, governor of Puerto Rico.

One award that must have appealed to Dr. Roberts's sense of fun was a membership certificate for the Guinea Pig Club of the Quartermaster Corps Subsistence Research and Development Laboratory. New members were greeted in doggerel:

Because you have now tasted and tested our grub
You've become a full member of our Guinea Pig Club.
By the use of the spoon you have brightened the light
For the search of those foods that help soldiers to fight.

Each of these awards was accompanied, of course, by a suitable citation. The tribute that seems to sum them up best was engraved on the plaque given her at the time she received the Marjorie Hulsizer Copher Award. It was written by Thelma E. Porter, who received her doctorate under Dr. Roberts's guidance, and who succeeded her as chairman of the Department of Home Economics at the University of Chicago:

> *Lydia Jane Roberts, in recognition of a distinguished leader and teacher of human nutrition; exponent of the ideals of The American Dietetic Association; pioneer in the development of nutrition work with children; and outstanding contributor to the establishment of sound national and international policies concerning nutrition. Her unusual ability to interpret scientific information and to devise methods of applying the principles of nutrition to human needs has led to the improvement of human welfare. Because of her broad interest and ambitious spirit, many have been inspired to follow her leadership.*[4]

Honors and tributes continued after Dr. Roberts's death. Dr. Jaime Benítez, Chancellor of the University of Puerto Rico, commemorated her in his commencement address in 1965, describing her as *"un cuerpo de paz y un alma en paz"* (a Peace Corps and a soul at peace). Memorial resolutions were passed in her honor by the American Home Economics Association and by the Food and Nutrition Board of the National Research Council. The members of the Puerto Rico Home Economics Association dedicated their annual meeting to her in June 1965.

In 1966 the first Lydia J. Roberts Memorial Lecture took place at the University of Puerto Rico, with Dr. William J. Darby as the speaker. These lectures have continued on a yearly basis since that time. In 1981 a Lydia J. Roberts Memorial Lecture Series was established by the University of Chicago Committee on Human Nutrition and Nutritional Biology. This lectureship, in which there is a yearly presentation by a distinguished nutritionist, is supported by a grant from the Quaker Oats Company.

Perhaps one of the greatest tributes to Lydia Roberts's memory has been the concern her associates have felt to finish her work. In her early years of research, she and her graduate students had gathered considerable data on food intake and growth of children. Dr. Roberts had always felt that these data should be combined and published—there was nothing comparable in the literature. She had gathered together the data and the theses related to the topic, and had all the material stored in the Blackstone Avenue apartment, where her sister Lil still lived. She also had talked with Bernice Wait Wood, a friend and former student who had helped to collect some of the original data, and had asked for her help. Dr. Roberts intended to work on the project when she left San Juan, but in the meantime Bernice Wood could get started on it. After Dr. Roberts's death, Bernice Wood, herself in her 80s, felt impelled to finish the project. She lived in the Blackstone Avenue apartment with Lillian Roberts for some time, organizing and summarizing the material. The results appeared in two papers in the *American Journal of Clinical Nutrition* in 1969 and 1973.[5,6]

In Puerto Rico, friends felt the same compelling urge to complete Lydia Roberts's work in that country. *Nutrición*, the Spanish-language textbook that Dr. Roberts was working on at the time of her death, was published in 1981.[7] The original material prepared by Dr. Roberts was updated, translated, and adapted for Puerto Rico by Rosa Marina Torres with the collaboration of the nutrition faculty of the School of Home Economics at the University of Puerto Rico. The book bears the name of Lydia J. Roberts as author.

The recognition that came to Lydia Roberts in her lifetime must have been a source of satisfaction. However, her pleasure was always tempered with humility and with an appreciation of the contributions of others. After she received the Field Award, she wrote to a friend who had been involved in preparing the presentation to the Field Foundation, "I appreciate it mostly because of your interest and friendship, and that of my friends who managed to assemble such a good array of evidence for me. That is the real satisfaction I get from it."

One of the most telling examples of Dr. Roberts's attitude toward success and praise can be found in a letter she wrote shortly after the 1962 publication of her book recounting the accomplishments of the community development project in Doña Elena. She told of the acknowledgments of the book that she had received:

> *All are pleased to have it, but only a few had read it. A few, however, had. One was McCollum. He. . . commented favorably on it, and also added a flattering comment about yours truly. . . . Dr. Robert Williams had also read it. . . . He had very complimentary things to say about it and me, among them hoping I'd live to be 120! So I could continue working on similar problems. . . . M. L. Wilson wrote another choice statement. I had written in the flyleaf recognition that he had first sent me to P.R. and got me involved in its affairs. He wrote "if I had something to do with your going to Puerto Rico, then I am justified in my pride in believing that it is the best job of its kind in the whole world." Imagine! I'm not telling these things to brag, merely taking courage from them.*

This, then, was Lydia Jane Roberts, a small-town girl from Michigan who achieved international recognition for her work in the fields of child nutrition and applied nutrition. She was just plain "Aunt Lyd" or "Lyd" to her family or Michigan friends, many of whom had no idea of the extent of her accomplishments, or "Miss Roberts," "Dr. Roberts," "Dr. Lydia," or "La Doctora" to her students and colleagues who, in contrast, marveled at her achievements. Variously described as a "people person" or a "private person," she was full of contrasts. She was a person of boundless energy and enthusiasm who bubbled over in her description of a sunset, a good meal, a concert, a party at a friend's house or at the governor's mansion, but a person who knew what is was like to be discouraged and frustrated. She had a passion for scientific accuracy and detail, but she also wanted that scientific knowledge applied for the good of humanity. She was a teacher all her life, whether in an elementary school in Montana, a university classroom, or an isolated village in Puerto Rico. She could empathize with the plights of undernourished children, and who worked, in a practical way, to feed them better. Her sense of humor carried her over the rough places, and her attitude toward life is best summed up by her comment: "As usual, I have too many irons in the fire. But it is more fun than not to have enough."

REFERENCES

1. Maretzki A: Where Every Prospect Pleases. Unpublished manuscript, 1978.
2. Bing FJ: Lydia J. Roberts—a biographical sketch. *J Nutr* 93:1, 1967.

3. *Lydia J. Roberts Award Essays: A Compilation of Essays.* Chicago, The American Dietetic Association, 1968.
4. Lydia J. Roberts receives 1952 Marjorie Hulsizer Copher Award. *J Am Diet Assoc* 28:1151, 1952.
5. Wait B, Blair R, Roberts LJ: Energy intakes of well-nourished children and adolescents. *Am J Clin Nutr* 22:1383, 1969.
6. Wait B: Protein intake of well-nourished children and adolescents. *Am J Clin Nutr* 26:1303, 1973.
7. Roberts LJ: *Nutrición.* San Juan, University of Puerto Rico, 1981.

CHAPTER 2

From Michigan to Montana to the Midway

Even though Lydia Roberts always had a warm spot in her heart for Martin, Michigan, apparently she decided quite early in her life that it was not the place in which she wanted to settle down forever. In retrospect, this does not seem surprising. The years of Lydia's growing up were important ones for women. By 1900, when she was starting her life's work, the idea of a woman seeking an education, a career, and independence was becoming acceptable—but it did represent a major change.

Although in this country beginning levels of schooling had been available for all since the early days of colonization, in the early part of the 19th century higher education was limited to an elite few who could afford it. Women who had attended elementary school and who had received training in the household arts from their mothers were considered well educated. There even seems to have been a general feeling that women were not educable beyond this point!

The tide was turning, however. By the middle of the 19th century a number of schools for the higher education of women had been established. Many of them were of the "finishing school" type, although some, such as Emma Willard, in Troy, New York, offered courses in housewifery. Women's colleges such as Mount Holyoke, founded in 1837, and Vassar, founded in 1861, offered liberal-arts education. These latter institutions, along with Smith, Wellesley, and other women's colleges of the same period, prided themselves on the fact that their curricula were comparable to those of the men's colleges—proving that women were indeed educable. In 1862 the Morrill Act, which established the land-grant colleges, was passed. The idea of education of women was sufficiently advanced by that time for some of these colleges to be coeducational, as were some other universities.[1] College education, for either sex, was still far from commonplace in the latter half of the 19th century, however. Only about 4% of the population between the ages of 18 and 25 attended college in 1900.[2]

Nevertheless, by the time Lydia Roberts finished high school in 1898, women were seeking college educations in steadily increasing numbers. Some women were abandoning the traditional women's colleges in favor of coeducational universities. In Boston, the Women's Collegiate Alumnae Association (later to become the American Association of University Women) had been formed in 1882. It is interesting to know that one of the first tasks of this new organization was a study of the health of women students, undertaken to dispel a popular notion that women were not physically capable of withstanding the rigors of higher education.[3] A few women had even stormed the traditional male strongholds of medicine and the law. The first woman to receive the degree of Doctor of Philosophy in this country, Helen Magill (White), graduated from Boston University in 1877.

When Lydia Roberts graduated from Martin High School her goal was to become an elementary-school teacher, and she enrolled in the Mount Pleasant Normal School (now Central Michigan University) in Mount Pleasant, Michigan. Today it is only a few hours' drive from Martin to Mount Pleasant, but in the days when Lydia was a student it must have been a real journey. It was still a new thing for a girl from a middle-class family to graduate from high school and go away to college. Only one with a lot of ambition and a lot of self-confidence would embark on such a program. In June of 1899, just a few days before her 20th birthday, Lydia received a Limited Teaching Certificate. This certificate was granted after a full academic year of work, and entitled the holder to teach in any rural school in the state. Teaching in elementary school became Lydia's occupation. There is no doubt that she liked it and was an enthusiastic and able teacher. Many years later, when working on nutrition projects, she was always delighted when she had the opportunity to work directly with children.

In the early years of the 20th century there was a demand for teachers in the rapidly growing towns of the western United States. This appealed to Lydia's adventurous spirit and desire for travel, and she left Michigan to teach in Montana. If Lydia's parents were concerned about her going so far from home, they probably were reassured by the fact that two of Warren Roberts's brothers had moved "out West" some time before—there was family in that part of the world. Lydia taught in both Miles City and Great Falls, Montana. She returned to the Midwest for a while, and completed work for her second teaching certificate. The Life Certificate was usually awarded after two years of training beyond high school. Persons holding it were qualified to teach in any elementary school, rural or urban. After receiving the Life Certificate in 1909, Lydia went back to Montana to the town of Dillon, where she taught third grade. In addition to her job as an elementary-school teacher, she also acted as a critic teacher for the normal school in Dillon, now known as Western Montana State College.

Apparently it was during the years in Dillon that Lydia Roberts began to make observations that were to lead her into a new career. As a good teacher she was interested not only in the education of her pupils, but also in their health and development. She was troubled to see children who she felt were not growing and developing satisfactorily. Her first real concern in this area came about as a result of summer work she had done in a children's institution in Montana. According to her sister, Lillian Roberts, as recounted to Dr. Franklin Bing, observations made that summer led Lydia to want to know more about the relationship between diet and health.[4] Perhaps the children in the institution where she worked seemed different from the children outside—listless, perhaps, or lethargic. Perhaps the food served in the institution was different from that eaten by healthy youngsters living with their own families. It is possible that once having started on this series of observations, she went beyond the institution to include observations of other children she saw in rural or small-town schools.

In the early 1900s Montana was still the frontier, and it is possible that some of the problems there were more acute than they were in more populated areas. Throughout the country, however, it was the custom at that time for many children attending rural or small-town schools to bring their lunches from home. These lunches, which usually consisted of a sandwich of meat and bread and a piece of pie or cake, were probably adequate in calories in most instances, but lacking in other nutrients provided by fruits and vegetables. Few, if any, children brought milk or other beverages from home. For most farm families of that period, the main meal of the day was at noon, and during the school year children missed that meal. In many cases, a sort of smorgasbord of leftovers from the noon meal served as the evening supper. It was from this somewhat limited assortment that a child had to make both his or her evening meal and, probably, his or her next day's lunch. Quite possibly, the diets of many of those children would be considered inadequate according to current standards—but at that time the importance of the *quality* as well as of the *quantity* of the food consumed was only beginning to be discovered.

Whatever observations Lydia Roberts had made, it is significant that she equated the food intake of the children with their health problems. Between 1910 and 1915, the science of nutrition was in its infancy. The growing discipline of organic chemistry had increased the knowledge of the nature of proteins, fats, and carbohydrates. The importance of certain minerals was recognized. Since about 1890, the work of Atwater and Benedict had made important contributions to the knowledge of energy metabolism and requirements. In 1906 Sir Frederick Gowland Hopkins, addressing the Academy of Science in London, had postulated that there was in food some as-yet-unknown substance (or substances) present in extremely small amounts that was essential for normal growth and development. His statement was based on a growing body of evidence from a variety of studies in different parts of the world.

Following Hopkins's statement, pieces of what seemed like a giant jigsaw puzzle began to fit into place. In 1912, Casimir Funk propounded the theory that beriberi, scurvy, pellagra, and possibly rickets were caused by a deficiency or lack in the diet of special substances that "are of the nature of organic bases, which we will call vitamines."[5] The new concept of dietary deficiency diseases was widely accepted. As work progressed, however, it became apparent that a variety of substances of different chemical types might be involved. The word *vitamine* was changed to *vitamin,* retaining the idea of a life-sustaining compound, but divorcing it from association with any particular chemical makeup. Starting in 1913, with the discovery of fat-soluble vitamin A, by E. V. McCollum at the University of Wisconsin, research in this new field was extensive and productive.

How much Lydia Roberts knew of these discoveries we do not know. As an intelligent person of lively curiosity and a wide variety of interests, she probably did have some knowledge of them. Even before the discovery of vitamins, which greatly stimulated public interest, women's magazines had begun to supplement recipes and meal plans with articles on nutrition. *Good Housekeeping,* for instance, had an article nearly every month, some of them by individuals such as Mary Davies Swartz (later Rose) of Columbia University[6] and John R. Murlin of Cornell,[7] who would become known as outstanding nutrition scientists. The topic of school lunch was also receiving a lot of attention at that time. Innovative school-lunch programs, menus for lunches brought from home, and the possibility of supplementing home-prepared lunches with milk or a hot dish at school were among the subjects addressed in women's magazines of the time.

Clearly nutrition was of interest, and information was reaching the public. The problem of how nutrition related to child well-being was Lydia Roberts's particular concern. This concern probably led her to read some of the child-growth studies that were appearing at the time. Beginning with the work of Bowditch in 1872, a number of researchers had begun to study growth patterns of children in different parts of the country, and to equate them with, among other things, differences in food intake. Although the findings of these studies were published in journals that probably were not readily available to an elementary-school teacher in Montana, there are some she might have seen. *Physical Growth and School Progress* by B. T. Baldwin,[8] published in 1914 as a bulletin of the US Bureau of Education, might easily have come to her attention. Baldwin reported that boys and girls who were tall and had good lung capacity were older physiologically and further along toward mental maturity as evidenced by school progress than were short, light boys and girls. This may have seemed to fit in with Lydia Roberts's own observations.

Whatever the reason, Lydia Roberts apparently became convinced that there was a relationship between the health status of the children she observed and their food intake. Characteristically, she decided she wanted to do something about the health of these children. Equally characteristically, she decided that if she were to be effective in her help, she must first know more about the relationship of diet and health—a decision that led, in 1915, to her enrollment in the University of Chicago, and to a new career.

Why Lydia Roberts chose the University of Chicago is another question that cannot be answered. Once she decided to seek further training, it would be characteristic of her to do some careful searching for the best place to go. Early in the decision process she probably came to the conclusion that the developing discipline of home economics was where she could get the kind of information she needed. No doubt she had read of the work of Ellen H. Richards, who played an outstanding role in the development of home economics in the United States.

Ellen Richards—then Ellen Swallow—had graduated from Vassar in 1870. Later that same year she received special permission to enter the Massachusetts Institute of Technology as a student in chemistry. In 1873 she received the Bachelor of Science degree, the first, and for some time, the only woman to be so honored by MIT. Married in 1875 to Professor R. H. Richards, a professor of mining engineering at MIT, she continued to work at the institute until her death in 1911.[2] Ellen Richards's interests lay in the field of "sanitary chemistry." The application of chemistry to the improvement of living conditions was of paramount importance to her, but the broadening and opening of the field of science to women was another engrossing interest. The melding of these two fields of interest was significant to her leading role in the development of the home economics movement.

It was largely through Ellen Richards's efforts that the first Lake Placid Conference was held in 1899. The purpose of the conference, as of subsequent ones, was to study "economic and social programs of the home, and problems of right living." It was at this first conference that the name *home economics* came into being.[1] Coincidentally, in the same year, Lydia Roberts was starting her own work in another field.

Lydia Roberts would have had no problem in getting information about programs in home economics from either the public press or university catalogs. Throughout 1910, when Lydia Roberts was first questioning the relationship between child health and food intake, and perhaps considering further training, *Good Housekeeping* had run a series of detailed articles on "home science" courses offered in the different states. Other information was no doubt available also. Certainly she had many choices. Most state universities, including Michigan State University in Lansing (not far from her home in Martin), were offering courses in home economics. However, if Lydia Roberts investigated the options thoroughly—as she probably did—she would have discovered that some of the most advanced work in home economics was being done at the University of Chicago under the leadership of Katharine Blunt in the Department of Home Economics and Marion Talbot in the Department of Household Administration. The article in *Good Housekeeping* on "Home Science Courses in Illinois" described the University of Chicago course as "most complete. . . and the very highest standards maintained. . . . Full college credit is given to the students, the same as those accorded to the students in Latin, Hebrew or Greek."[9]

In making her decision, Lydia Roberts undoubtedly examined many university catalogs. From the *University of Chicago Register* she would have learned that graduate as well as undergraduate work was being offered in both the Departments of Home Economics and of Household Administration. Indeed, the first PhD in this new field had been carried out under Marion Talbot's direction, and had been granted to Edna Day (Hyde) in 1906.[10] In 1915 Lydia Roberts still had to complete her bachelor's degree,but even then, in the back of her mind at least, she might have been considering the advantages of advanced study.

Whatever Lydia Roberts's reasons for choosing the then-young University of Chicago, there is no doubt that when she arrived on the Midway, she found herself in a challenging atmosphere, one that must have had much appeal to a person of her background and capabilities. She had also found what was to be her academic home for the next 30 years.

REFERENCES

1. Craig HT: *The History of Home Economics.* New York, Practical Home Economics, 1945, pp 5,9.
2. East M: *Home Economics, Past, Present and Future.* Boston, Allyn and Bacon, 1980, pp 44,45.
3. Talbot M: *More than Lore.* Chicago, University of Chicago Press, 1936, p 145.
4. Bing FJ: Lydia Jane Roberts—a biographical sketch. *J Nutr* 93:1, 1967.
5. McCollum EV: *History of Nutrition.* Boston, Houghton Mifflin Co, 1957, p 217.

6. Swartz MD: How much meat? *Good Housekeeping*, January 1910, p 106.
7. Murlin JR: The training table. II Food requirements for moderate work; III Food requirements for muscular work; IV Food requirements for brain work. *Good Housekeeping*, January, February, March 1911, pp 102, 248, 349.
8. Baldwin BT: *Physical Growth and School Progress*. Bulletin no. 10. Washington, DC, US Bureau of Education, 1914.
9. Kirkwood EB: Home science in Illinois. *Good Housekeeping*, October 1910, p 602.
10. Dye M: *Home Economics at the University of Chicago, 1892–1956*. Chicago, University of Chicago Home Economics Alumni Association, 1972, p 216.

CHAPTER 3

Chicago, a Fertile Environment

Although known today for excellence in basic rather than applied disciplines, the University of Chicago, in its first 50 years, played a major role in the development of home economics in the United States. Lydia Roberts was an important contributor in this development.

When Lydia Roberts came to the University of Chicago in 1915, it was a new school, barely 25 years old. Incorporated in 1890, the university held its first classes in 1892. By 1915 it was already known as a "different" university. The programs in home economics and in household administration were different, too, with their stress on both graduate studies, and learning, through strong work in basic sciences, the "whys" as well as the "hows." The environment was ideal for a mature, goal-oriented student such as Lydia.

The vitality and excitement of the University of Chicago was due in large part to the energy and enthusiasm of its first president, Dr. William Rainey Harper. Dr. Harper had strong convictions as to what he thought a university should be. He had accepted the presidency of the University of Chicago only after he had sold its founders on his concept of a graduate research school on an equal footing with the undergraduate college.[1]

Once appointed, in 1891, Harper turned his amazing energies to gathering the best faculty possible. He lured distinguished members of long-established university faculties with promises of larger salaries. Bright young people of promise came because of the opportunities for scholarship and research. Raising additional funds to support such a program became an important part of Harper's new job, as was the supervision of the construction of the university buildings in the Hyde Park area of the city's south side, along the famous Midway of the Columbian Exposition.

Among the outstanding faculty who opened the university was Marion Talbot, a young woman from Boston. She and another New Englander, Alice Peloubet Norton, who would come to the university a decade later, were largely responsible for the early development of what would eventually become the Department of Home Economics and Household Administration. Both of these women had a close association in their student years with Ellen H. Richards.

Marion Talbot came from a distinguished New England family. Her father was dean of the Medical School of Boston University. Her mother was active in the social and community activities of Boston. Marion graduated from Boston University in 1880 and went on to study for a master's degree, which she received in 1882.[2] During her graduate study, she also became involved in an activity that would interest her for the rest of her life, a union of women who had graduated from college.

The initial development of this new interest is described by Marion Talbot in her autobiography, *More than Lore*: "I consulted with Mrs. Ellen H. Richards, who had graduated from Vassar College in 1870, and was teaching at the Massachusetts Institute of Technology. We summoned for conference, the few college women we knew. . .and in 1882, the Association of Collegiate Alumnae was formed."[2]

The Association of Collegiate Alumnae went on to become the American Association of University Women, an organization in which Marion Talbot played an active role for many years. As a part of her activities in the early years of the organization, Marion Talbot became a member, in 1885, of a Sanitary Science Club, with Ellen Richards as leader. Alice Peloubet, a graduate of Smith College, was also a member. The association with Ellen Richards in the club proved to be important for these young women.

Through their work in the Sanitary Science Club, both Marion Talbot and Alice Peloubet were influenced by the dynamic Ellen Richards to become interested in studies on the welfare of the home and household. Both of them would go on to study with Ellen Richards at MIT. Both were participants in the Lake Placid Conferences, which were continued, on an invitation-only basis, from 1899 to 1909. By 1909, when the American Home Economics Association was formed with Ellen Richards as its first president, both Marion Talbot and Alice Peloubet were members of the University of Chicago faculty.[3]

Marion Talbot entered MIT shortly after the founding of the Sanitary Science Club and received the degree of Bachelor of Science in 1888. Following her graduation, she was a lecturer at the Lasell Seminary in Boston, and in 1890 she was appointed instructor in domestic science at Wellesley.[2] The president of Wellesley at the time of Marion Talbot's appointment to the faculty was Alice Freeman Palmer, who had also been a founding member of the Collegiate Alumnae Association. Alice Palmer was one of the faculty brought to the new University of Chicago by William Rainey Harper. It was through Alice Palmer's recommendation that Marion Talbot received an offer from President Harper to become assistant professor of

Sanitary Science and Dean of Women (undergraduate). Since there was to be no department of domestic science in the university, the courses taught by Marion Talbot were to be included in the Department of Social Science.

Marion Talbot lost no time in making her mark at the new university, not only in her own field, but in the whole area of the education of women. She thought that most women could benefit from preparation for more efficient homemaking—or "household administration," as she called it—as a part of their college educations. Since college was taking an increasing number of women out of the home during the years when they might otherwise have been learning housekeeping skills, this training had considerable appeal to many girls and their parents. In Marion Talbot's view, such training should be more than "cooking and sewing." She was a firm believer in the importance of a good general education and in a solid foundation in the basic sciences. Marion Talbot also fully concurred with President Harper's concern for the importance of graduate work. From 1893 onward, the space devoted to Sanitary Science in the *University of Chicago Register* listed courses required for graduate study, as well as courses for which graduate credit was given.

In 1904 the Section of Sanitary Science became the Department of Household Administration, with Marion Talbot as its head. One of the faculty members of the new department was Sophanisba T. Breckenridge. Sophanisba Breckenridge held a doctorate in political science, and was also a graduate of the University of Chicago School of Law, the first woman to take its JD degree.

According to Marion Talbot, the home at the beginning of the century

> *. . . was rapidly becoming a consuming rather than a producing center. This called for less study of methods of domestic manufacturing, and more study of those industrial and governmental institutions through whose agency the householder is enabled to care more effectively for her family and household. Dr. Breckenridge offered courses. . . [such as] "Standards of Child Care"; "Legal and Economic Position of Women"; "Care of Families in Distress"; while I offered "The House as a Factor in Health"; together with courses on the social, economic, hygienic and legal aspects of dietetics and the administration of the modern household.*[2]

In many ways the new Department of Household Administration, with its emphasis on these types of subject matter, was a forerunner of the family-oriented home economics programs of today—perhaps, as Marion Talbot speculated in her autobiography, it was "ahead of the times."

By the time that the new Department of Household Administration was a reality, a Department of Home Economics had also come into existence in the university. This department was located in the School of Education, which had been established in 1901 with Col. F. W. Parker, former director of the Chicago Institute, as its head. The Home Economics Department was an outgrowth of courses in "domestic economy" that had been offered in the University Laboratory School as a part of John Dewey's experiments on "learning by doing," and of two courses that had been offered in the Department of Pedagogy, which were essentially concerned with teaching methods in domestic arts.[3] The initial function of the new department was primarily to train teachers of home economics.

Colonel Parker brought Alice Peloubet Norton with him to the University of Chicago. Alice Peloubet had married Professor Lewis Norton of the chemistry department at MIT. His death left her a young widow with small children and led her to decide to fit herself for a teaching career. She followed Marion Talbot's example and enrolled at MIT, where she worked under Ellen Richards's guidance. When Colonel Parker approached Ellen Richards for someone to inaugurate work in home economics at the Chicago Institute, she recommended Alice Norton.[3]

Thus it came about that Marion Talbot and Alice Norton, friends of many years, with similar backgrounds and many similar ideas on education, found themselves at the same university, but in separate departments. When the Department of Household Administration was formed, Alice Norton was asked to teach the courses in foods that involved laboratory experimentation. As Alice Norton wrote later, this "brought about a certain unification of the two departments, but introduced administrative problems that were sometimes difficult."[4] The two departments continued as separate entities for some 20 years.

Alice Peloubet Norton left the University of Chicago in 1913 to become editor of the *Journal of Home Economics.* In that same year, Katharine Blunt was appointed assistant professor in the Department of Home Economics, and six years later, in 1919, she became its head. Dr. Blunt also was an Easterner, from Philadelphia. She graduated from Vassar in 1898 with a major in chemistry. She also had spent a year in advanced study at MIT. She received her doctorate in chemistry from the University of Chicago in 1907.[3]

Under Dr. Blunt's direction, emphasis on research and graduate study in the Department of Home Economics increased, and by 1919, when she became its head, three doctorates had been granted. During the ten years of Dr. Blunt's chairmanship, 17 more PhDs and 163 master's were granted. In a 1925 report to the President of the University, Dr. Blunt pointed out that the University of Chicago was the only university in the United States offering the PhD in home economics and that only one other university in the country granted as many master's degrees in that field as Chicago.[3]

In addition to the thriving graduate program, undergraduate enrollment increased during this period, and there were approximately 20 faculty members. Work was offered in the fields of food and nutrition, institution economics, household arts, textiles and related arts, home economics education, household management, and child development.

With her background in elementary education, it is not surprising that Lydia Roberts chose the Department of Home Economics in the School of Education as her academic home. When she came to the university in 1915, the department was vigorous and growing rapidly. Although, at age 36, she was older than most students, she undoubtedly felt the vitality, excitement, and challenge that students at the University of Chicago still experience today. In her mentor, Katharine Blunt (only a few years older than she), Lydia Roberts found a friend and a challenging example to follow. And, most important, she found her true vocation. The study of nutrition and its application for human betterment provided a fitting outlet for her intellectual abilities and for her unbounding energy and enthusiasm. As a successful elementary teacher she had a deep interest in and love for children, and a concern for their welfare. Her new profession enabled her to express this concern in concrete, practical ways. The area of child nutrition was to be a major interest throughout her professional life.

Although Lydia Roberts was admitted to the university with advanced standing, it is doubtful that her normal-school training had given her the science background she would need for her new field. She must have had to start with the basics. According to the *University of Chicago Register* for 1915–16, requirements for the bachelor's degree in home economics included courses in inorganic and organic chemistry, mathematics, and physics, as well as courses in home economics and in education. Recommended electives included courses in political economy, political science, psychology, sociology, bacteriology, and qualitative and quantitative analysis.[5] Although Lydia Roberts was interested in children, there were no courses in child nutrition for her to take—she was the one who would later develop and present them. In spite of the rigorous program she must have followed, Lydia Roberts completed the work for the Bachelor of Philosophy degree in two years—and completed it brilliantly, for she was admitted to membership in Phi Beta Kappa.

It is likely that when Lydia Roberts came to the University of Chicago, she had expected to return to Montana to put her new knowledge to practical use. In the new atmosphere in which she found herself, however, it probably was not difficult for her to change her mind and stay in Chicago. For one thing, the country was at war. Many army draftees had been found to be in poor physical condition, and it was thought that poor food habits were to blame in many cases. Public interest in food and nutrition was at a peak. Clearly, additional study for a master's degree would be advantageous.

Particularly appealing to the new graduate was a project just getting under way at the university. Dr. Blunt had worked out an arrangement in 1917 with the directors of the Central Free Dispensary of Rush Medical College to enable home economics graduate students to work directly with children. Lydia Roberts's excellent scholastic record, together with her experience as an elementary-school teacher, gave her ideal qualifications for carrying out an important part of the project—developing a nutrition-education program for children in the clinic.[6] So in 1917, Lydia Roberts embarked on her second career when she was appointed instructor in the Department of Home Economics of the University of Chicago. The work in the clinic was a major part of her responsibilities, and developing the children's nutrition program constituted the work for her master's thesis. She received the degree of Master of Science in 1918. Her thesis was published in the *Journal of Home Economics* in 1919,[7] the first of her many published papers on child nutrition.

In 1919, after completing her degree and publishing her thesis, Lydia Roberts was promoted to the rank of assistant professor in the Department of Home Economics. She taught several courses and had a variety of responsibilities in the department, but her major interest continued to be in the field of child nutrition. She developed and taught the first course in this field to be offered in the department. She also was closely involved with the Cooperative Nursery School at the University of Chicago as its adviser on nutrition and, starting in 1925, as a member of its board of directors. The relationship between the Department of Home Economics and the nursery school was close and cordial for many years, affording students the opportunity for observation and practice, for research, and for developing innovative teaching techniques. During several summer quarters in the 1920s, the Department of Home Economics emphasized work in child study with systematic observations in the nursery school. In these programs Lydia Roberts offered courses in diet for children, child care, and nutrition work with children; other experts offered work in the psychological study of children.

In addition to teaching, research, and extensive committee work at both the local and national level, Lydia Roberts continued to take university courses and to gather material for her PhD dissertation. One of the students in the department during this period recalled, "Miss Roberts had a great desire for knowledge. I recall her writing me about taking a year's course in physiology in the medical school . . . that was a hard course and took great determination and desire. Imagine lab work after a day of teaching!"

Work on her doctorate proceeded slowly—but with all Lydia Roberts's activities, how could it be otherwise? In 1928, ten years after she had received the master's degree, her PhD was granted. The event was noted by her promotion to associate professor. She was elected to membership in Sigma Xi in the same year. A year earlier, the University of Chicago Press had published her entire dissertation as a book, *Nutrition Work With Children*.[8] This book was destined to become known as a masterpiece in nutrition literature.

Publication of *Nutrition Work With Children* marked an important milestone in nutrition education. It was the first text or reference book devoted entirely to child nutrition. Its purpose, as stated by Dr. Roberts in the book's foreword, was "to present the problem of malnutrition as it affects childhood, together with practical methods for its eradication."

Nutrition Work With Children had been developed as a textbook for a course bearing the same name, which Lydia Roberts had taught since 1919. It is significant that while the book included a complete review of the literature on child nutrition at that time, the greatest number of references in the extensive bibliography had been published within the previous ten years. In 1927, the nutrition movement was essentially new. Relatively few publications on child nutrition had appeared prior to 1917; the number increased dramatically, however, in the following years.

The first half of the book dealt primarily with the nature, causes, and effects of malnutrition, and with standards for normal nutrition. The second half dealt with methods of prevention and treatment of malnutrition through nutrition work in schools, infant welfare clinics, nursery schools, and other agencies reaching preschool children. In the second part Dr. Roberts stressed the importance of nutrition education in schools, an idea she would continue to advocate throughout her career.

In 1929, Lydia Roberts, a new PhD at age 50, was about to enter another phase of her career. Dr. Katharine Blunt resigned in that year to become president of Connecticut College for Women. A steering committee was appointed to find a new department head. In addition to being a member of the committee, Dr. Roberts was named acting head of the Department of Home Economics. It was a time of change and reorganization in the university, and the committee's work proceeded slowly.

In April 1930, the American Institute of Nutrition held its annual meeting in Chicago. Among those in attendance were a number of alumnae of the University of Chicago Department of Home Economics. They were concerned that an appointment to replace Dr. Blunt had not yet been made. In the opinion of these alumnae, one person was ideally suited to fill the vacant position, and that was Lydia J. Roberts, the acting head. These alumnae drafted a letter to President Robert

Maynard Hutchins strongly recommending Dr. Roberts's appointment. Certainly her credentials were impressive. In the years that she had been a member of the faculty of the university, she had not only completed her doctorate and published a major nutrition text, but had conducted extensive research. Her publications had included papers in scientific journals, two major bulletins for the Children's Bureau, and a wide variety of papers on nutrition for teachers and for the lay public. She had served, or was serving, on important national committees having to do with child nutrition (including three committees of the White House Conference on Children, which met in 1929). She had developed a number of innovative educational programs and had proved herself to be an effective teacher, researcher, and administrator.

The letter recommending Dr. Roberts was signed by some 30 people and was followed by letters from Dr. Blunt and a number of other individuals familiar with Dr. Roberts's work, all urging the appointment. President Hutchins was convinced and announced Lydia Roberts's appointment, subject to the approval of the board of trustees in June. The appointment was confirmed, and at the same time Dr. Roberts was promoted to the rank of professor.

Probably Dr. Roberts was well aware that she would be facing difficult problems in her new job. Some of them had already become apparent during the last years of Dr. Blunt's administration. Although the department's growth had been rapid during Katharine Blunt's tenure, it had not been without difficulties. A major problem was limited space. In 1903, when Emmons Blaine Hall was built, the Department of Home Economics had been assigned quarters in the new building. These doubtless seemed adequate, even spacious, at that time. But the University Laboratory School, which was also housed in Blaine Hall, had expanded, too. No more space had been made available to the department.

In 1924 Marion Talbot retired from the university. The Department of Household Administration was merged with the Department of Home Economics to form the Department of Home Economics and Household Administration in the College of Arts and Sciences. The joining of Marion Talbot's concepts for training with the dynamic leadership of Katharine Blunt created a fine department—a "different" department—but, unfortunately, it did not result in any additional space. In fact, it was only intervention by the dean of the College of Education that kept the department in Blaine Hall. Following the merger, Dr. Blunt submitted a major reorganization plan that included a statement of long-term financial needs. Strong attempts also were made to gain larger quarters, preferably in the form of a new building. In the rapidly growing university, however, funds were not available to solve the space needs of a small department, no matter how deserving. Attempts to raise funds from private sources were unsuccessful.[3] The department continued to get along with the same limited facilities for many years. Some have speculated that in some ways students felt challenged by these limitations and put forth extra efforts to produce quality research under both physical and financial limitations.

At the time Dr. Roberts assumed her new position, two major changes were occurring (in addition to these ongoing departmental problems) that would eventually affect the future of home economics at the University of Chicago. One of these was general in nature. Since the early years of the century, the large land-grant colleges, with their emphasis on the practical disciplines of engineering and agriculture, had been devoting increasing amounts of space and funds to home economics. With the more adequate space, equipment, and funding available in these colleges, as well as the quality staffs that were being formed, students were drawn to them in increasing numbers. University of Chicago graduates were prominent among the staff rosters of many of these growing home economics departments.

The other change was specific to the University of Chicago. In 1928, Robert Maynard Hutchins had become the new president of the university. This brilliant young man, only 29 years old at the time of his appointment, was to make the university famous with his innovative educational policies. The university was completely reorganized in the early years of his administration.

Under the new organizational plan, a University College was established, where students followed a program of general education for two years. After completing their college work and passing comprehensive examinations, they moved into one of four divisions (biological sciences, humanities, physical sciences, and social sciences) or into one of the professional schools.

Although this new organization had many advantages, it was difficult for an interdisciplinary department such as home economics. Students in the nutrition and food chemistry sections had their academic home in the Division of the Biological Sciences, those in family economics and in child development in the Division of the Social Sciences, those in textiles and related arts in the Division of the Humanities. Most of the students in the college, some of whom had entered after their second year of high school, knew little—and had little opportunity to learn—about the field of home economics. In many cases the University College students probably took an elitist view of home economics as dealing with "cooking and sewing." Undergraduate enrollment in the department dropped.

During the 15 years that Dr. Roberts was head of the Department of Home Economics and Household Administration, she continued the search for additional funds and for additional space. She also sought to reorganize the department in the more efficient form of a school or an institute of home economics.

According to Marie Dye, the historian of the Home Economics Department, "Records indicate that several administrators favored the formation of an 'Institute' or 'School of Home Economics,' but no action was taken."[3]

Despite the decline in undergraduate enrollment, graduate work in home economics continued to thrive. During the time that Lydia Roberts was chairman of the department, 36 PhDs and 208 master's degrees were granted. Of these, some 20 PhDs and 64 master's degrees were under the primary direction of Dr. Roberts.[3]

That the University of Chicago continued to maintain its reputation for excellence in graduate training in home economics was a credit to Dr. Roberts's leadership and administrative abilities. According to a former staff member, "She presented the Department of Home Economics to the University of Chicago administration with skill and tact. She encouraged and supported each member of the faculty of the department."

Dr. Roberts probably had many opportunities to move on to other positions during the time she was at the University of Chicago. Perhaps she gave serious consideration to some offers. Those who were associated with her, however, felt that despite the many problems that confronted her, she was completely dedicated to the Home Economics Department and to the University of Chicago and the tradition of excellence that it maintained. In this dedication she appears to have been joined by both faculty and students. Certainly for many graduate students in nutrition who came into the department during those years, first impressions were often a shock. Classroom and laboratory facilities were limited, especially when compared with those of the large land-grant and state universities that many of the students had attended as undergraduates. But few, if any, failed to fall under the spell of the dynamic Lydia Roberts, and few, if any, left the university feeling that their education or training was in any way inadequate.

In 1944 Dr. Roberts reached the age of 65, the mandatory retirement age at the University of Chicago at that time. She was not the kind of person who would regard retirement with much favor under any circumstances, but she must have felt a special sadness, retiring at the time she did, in leaving her successor, Thelma Porter, with so many unsolved problems. Some progress was made in dealing with these problems in the years immediately following World War II. In 1945 work was started on remodeling an apartment building at 5757 Drexel into classrooms and laboratories for the nutrition and food science sections, which were finally moved out of Blaine Hall. The move was completed in 1952. Laboratories and classrooms for textiles and related arts were moved to another remodeled apartment building at 5741 Drexel. The heads of the family economics and child development sections had their offices and student headquarters in the Departments of Economics and of Psychology, respectively. Although undergraduate enrollment was low, graduate students, especially at the doctoral level, continued to be attracted. During the 11 years of Thelma Porter's administration, 20 PhD degrees and 38 master's degrees were granted.[3]

In 1952 the Department of Home Economics became a Committee on Home Economics, with an advisory committee of six professors from different areas of the university where home economics students were involved. Although individual members of the committee were generally in sympathy with the importance of home economics as a fundamental field of learning, they failed

> *. . . to find a solution for the serious problem of Home Economics—adequate financial support and a place in the University organization that would permit Home Economics to grant degrees that would meet University requirements, but also meet the needs of its various fields.*[3]

As faculty retired or resigned, funds were not made available for their replacement. Finally, in 1956, President Lawrence Kimpton wrote a letter to the alumnae of the department, telling them of the committee's dissolution.

Even though there was not a place for home economics in the University of Chicago as it developed in the postwar years, the university program had made a major impact. The emphasis on solid education and on the importance of research, and the openness to new and innovative educational approaches all helped to produce a group of outstanding alumnae who did much to set the standards for later development in the field.

For Lydia Roberts, the healthy academic climate of the university from 1915 to 1944 provided a fertile environment for the development and growth of her own particular interests in nutrition.

> *My field of interest is human nutrition, especially child nutrition, in its public health and social welfare aspects. I recognize fully the necessity for fundamental research on animals and in the chemistry laboratory for determining the basic principles of nutrition, but I have chosen to devote my own efforts to the problem of interpreting nutrition in terms of human requirements and to devising ways and means by which the nutrition knowledge we now have may be utilized for human betterment.*[9]

This statement, the introduction to a report on "The Interests and Activities of Lydia J. Roberts," which was prepared in 1938, apparently in response to a university request, sums up the goals of Dr. Roberts's second career. Her standards for acquiring nutrition knowledge were rigorous. Students must be well grounded in basic science, and research must be well planned and well executed. For the knowledge gained to be truly significant, in her view, it should be broadly disseminated and used for human good. It is doubtful that any of the graduate students who came under her influence, whether in class, in seminars, or in research, ever failed to think of the practical implications of their own work or that of others. Certainly, Lydia Roberts's dedication to these ideas was an important factor in her success in teaching, research, and public service during the years she was at the University of Chicago.

REFERENCES

1. Mullin W: A meeting of minds. *Chicago Tribune* 29 September 1985, Sunday Magazine.
2. Talbot M: *More than Lore.* Chicago, University of Chicago Press, 1937, pp 144, 150.
3. Dye M: *Home Economics at the University of Chicago, 1892—1956.* Chicago, University of Chicago Home Economics Alumni Association, 1972, pp 58, 90, 105, 125, 128, 132.
4. Norton AP: Marion Talbot. *J Home Econ* 17:479, 1925.
5. *University of Chicago Register, 1915—16.*
6. Bing F J: Lydia J. Roberts—a biographical sketch. *J Nutr* 93:1, 1967.
7. Roberts LJ: A malnutrition clinic as a university problem in applied dietetics. *J Home Econ* 11:95, 1919.
8. Roberts LJ: *Nutrition Work With Children.* Chicago, University of Chicago Press, 1927.
9. Roberts LJ: Statement of Interests and Recent Activities of Lydia J. Roberts. Report on file. Chicago, University of Chicago Archives, 1938.

CHAPTER 4

Spreading the Gospel of Good Nutrition

I may be regarded, I suppose, as a "pioneer" in the field of nutrition work with children. In 1918 I organized a nutrition class for malnourished children and their parents in Central Free Dispensary of Rush Medical College, and utilized it also as field work for students of nutrition in the University of Chicago. . . . Since this early venture I have extended my interest to other avenues and methods through which nutritional improvement of children might be effected; nutrition education in the public school, in the school lunchroom, in the nursery school, and in other public health and welfare agencies. This has been effected mainly through teaching students of nutrition, who have gone out into schools, colleges, child welfare organizations, and other agencies and spread the gospel of good nutrition in the communities which they served.[1]

If Lydia Roberts had been asked to list her personal interests and priorities in the field of nutrition, improving child nutrition undoubtedly would have headed the list. It was the concern that had led her into the field of nutrition; it was a major concern throughout her professional career, even after she became involved in many additional aspects of nutrition science and education.

Not all of Dr. Roberts's students followed her footsteps into child nutrition. Their interests and later accomplishments were many and varied. That most of them joined the crusade to "spread the gospel" in their chosen fields was in great part due to Dr. Roberts's skill as a teacher—a teacher who not only taught, but inspired others to teach.

Even those who felt in awe of Lydia Roberts or who never felt close to her agreed that she was a gifted teacher. In class, students were impressed by the clarity of her presentation. They enjoyed her stories of nutrition "greats" whom she knew well, and they loved the humorous anecdotes with which she enlivened her lectures. When the quarter ended, they felt challenged by her well-written and thought-provoking examinations. If they had the opportunity to take part in one of her workshops, they were impressed with her creativity and her ability to make the subject relevant. If they had the good fortune to work with her on some project involving small children, they were struck by her skill in talking to and working with the children. New students were sometimes taken aback by the length of the reading lists they received on the first day of class—but later were surprised by how much they had read. It was just part of the challenge that many students reported they had felt in their contacts with Dr. Roberts, the challenge to really do their best.

Lydia Roberts's success as a teacher was due in part, of course, to the excellence of her presentation and to her expertise—"her vast nutrition knowledge" as one student put it. But her ability to inspire, to generate interest, went beyond that. Like most good teachers, she was deeply interested in her students. She had the ability to recognize their skills, to encourage them, to help them over rough spots, and to rejoice with them in their successes.

Sometimes Dr. Roberts's enthusiasm and her interest and concern were influential even before she had any personal contact with a student, but came about instead through a letter, a speech, or some of her publications. One student told of how, when she was considering graduate school,

> *I wrote letters to Home Economics departments in a number of universities, outlining my interests and requesting information. In due course I received catalogs from all of them, sometimes accompanied by a printed card or note. From Chicago, however, came a page-long letter from Miss Roberts, analyzing my particular situation, and answering my questions. I was impressed! So much so, in fact, that I decided then and there to go to Chicago—a good decision, and one I never regretted.*

A Puerto Rican student wrote:

> *I was [at the University of Puerto Rico] to study bacteriology. One day I was walking through the Home Economics School where Dr. Roberts was giving a lecture about the nutritional problems of the world, her words called my attention and I went in. What she said really amazed me, and I started to think about all the things that could be done to fight against this problem; after that I decided to study nutrition.*

Another student wrote of having been an elementary-school teacher in a part of the country that had suffered a severe economic setback. She was concerned about the children, who, she felt, had inadequate food and medical care.

> *In order to . . . try to learn what to do to help them, I enrolled in Home Economics. . . . During my senior year (1926—27) I realized I had not learned what I needed to know in order to help those children. But that winter I*

discovered a copy of Dr. Roberts' text book. . . . I determined to go to Chicago to study under her. Those years of 1928–30 were truly wonderful. . . . The Depression of the 1930s soon took its tolls. Again, there were starving children. But this time—thanks to my work with Dr. Roberts—I could be of some help to them and their families.

Good teachers generally have one trait in common: they are interested in their students, not only as recipients of the knowledge they have to impart, but as human beings. Dr. Roberts was no exception, and many letters commented on this facet of her teaching. However, some students never felt close to her. "I'm apologetic I have nothing to send you," wrote one person who had received her doctorate under Dr. Roberts's direction. "Even though I was her student, I didn't know her very well." Another person wrote, "When I got to know Dr. Roberts a little better. . . later, she seemed less formidable. I had been a bit scared of her as a student."

Many more letters, however, expressed appreciation for the help and encouragement the writers had received during their student years—help and encouragement that in many cases went far beyond the usual student-teacher-adviser relationship. Among the phrases used to describe Dr. Roberts were "kind and caring," "gentle," "fair," "sensitive," "understanding," "compassionate"—even "motherly." Some felt that she had actually influenced the course of their lives. "If it hadn't been for Dr. Roberts and her kindness and encouragement, I personally would not have had a University degree. . . I feel eternal gratitude to her."

A Puerto Rican colleague said she was sure she would never have finished her doctorate if it had not been for Dr. Roberts. She had neither finished writing her dissertation nor taken her final exams when she received a job offer in Puerto Rico that she could not resist. "Miss Roberts kept telling me and telling me I must finish," she recalled. "In the summer of 1944 she was going to be in Chicago. She said 'you're coming with me.' I stayed at her apartment; I worked night and day—and, thanks to Dr. Roberts, I finished!"

Other people wrote of the influence she had had on their professional lives. "I am convinced that my professional career was greatly enhanced by having worked with Dr. Roberts," one student wrote, while another reported, "At the University of Chicago I came under the tutelage and guidance of the one person who most influenced my professional life, Lydia J. Roberts. . . from my first contact with her, Lydia J. Roberts influenced me most because it was she who led me to believe that there was only one field worth pursuing for my life's work, and that was child nutrition."

For Lydia Roberts, teaching was not just a one-way process, however. She appreciated the stimulation and the response she got from her students and she often thanked them for it. In the letter one former student wrote, she enclosed a copy of a letter she had received from Dr. Roberts—a letter she had kept for nearly 40 years! Dr. Roberts had written, "Thank you for your words of appreciation . . . about your year here. I can assure you the appreciation was mutual. You were a very satisfactory, stimulating student, and I enjoyed very much having you in my classes."

Lydia Roberts's success as a teacher was not all based on personal charisma, or even on expertise. She was a teacher with high standards for herself and for the students. To gain her approval, students needed to work hard and perform well. Although they did not always enjoy the pressure, most students appreciated the results. "Dr. Roberts was exacting, her standards were high," one person wrote, "but she had a way of presenting her material so that one was willing to work beyond what was absolutely necessary." Another student commented on the "countless hours" she had spent in Crerar Library while she was in school, because "Dr. Roberts inspired me to read in a way that I had not done before." Another type of sentiment was expressed by the student who wrote, "We were always in awe of her, and had our assignments in on time and correct." Dr. Roberts could indeed be a stern critic at times. One person said, "I'll never forget when I turned in my proposal for my Master's thesis. She ripped it up and down! But, you know, it *wasn't* very good!" Presumably the next attempt was much better, for she went on to finish the degree, and to become an admirer of her critic.

Sometimes Dr. Roberts's encouragement of students took the form of a challenge. "She had groomed me for being a leader in the field of nutrition," one of her early students wrote, ". . . and I wasn't always quite sure whether I had nerve enough and imagination enough to do it. So she gave me opportunities that I wondered about . . . and then I did it because she asked it." A student who had married during the time she was working on a master's degree wrote:

> *. . . I got the distinct impression, though it was not said in so many words, that she thought I was a lost cause as a professional person. I have, therefore, spent the rest of my life endeavoring to prove to myself, to others, and to her (though she did not know it) that I could make a contribution in a professional area which later became known as community nutrition.*

Lydia Roberts believed in challenging students in other ways, too. Whenever possible, the broad facilities of the university were used in planning programs, and students found themselves taking courses in the departments of chemistry, biochemistry, physiology, and histology. Many of their classmates were medical students, and it was a source of pride that the women from Blaine Hall were able to hold their own. One student of the late 1920s wrote:

Dr. Roberts planned our programs so that we had courses under distinguished professors. I had work in Histology under Dr. Bensley and Dr. Bloom, Genetics under Dr. Newman, and Physiology under Dr. Carlson. To me the great challenge of studying at the University was that all my professors expected us to pursue our own interests in the subjects under study. . . [Weekends] found us in the libraries and laboratories hard at work. . . That delving into the new has kept me at my learning to this day.

Although there was no formal training in teaching techniques in Dr. Roberts's classes, students were never allowed to forget that in addition to being learners, they were also to be communicators. Her interest in "spreading the nutrition gospel" was so great that her students could not fail to realize that, no matter what kind of job they had, they would, in their turn, be passing on nutrition information. They were reminded of this in every classroom activity. Papers were criticized on the basis of organization and style as well as content. Answers on examinations were expected to be succinct and to the point. Spoken presentations, in classes or seminars, should be well organized and well presented.

Students were much aware of the emphasis on communication. "Dr. Roberts's class presentations were consistently well organized, logical and clear," one person wrote. "She insisted that we, as students, present our reports in similar fashion and I feel I owe to her the practice I have followed (for better or for worse) of planning and preparing in detail every public talk." Furthermore, reports should be not only clear, but interesting. Another student commented, "She insisted that, no matter how technical, we try to make the subject of a talk 'come alive' for our audience, but never at the expense of accuracy or level of understanding. She practiced that approach herself."

Any lessons in communication that Dr. Roberts gave were largely in the form of examples. She was a firm believer in the use of visual aids, both in her own presentations and in those of others. Scientific data, either from the literature or from original research, should be presented in a clear style and should be illustrated whenever possible by charts and graphs. These charts, if they were used in a class or seminar, should be not only intelligible, but legible from the back of the room. If other types of visual presentations were feasible and appropriate, they also should be used.

As far as Dr. Roberts was concerned, visual aids did not have to be elaborate or expensive. One of her Puerto Rican associates commented on her "ability to use simple, inexpensive, but very effective materials. She would make charts out of practically nothing. Wrapping paper, card board and Magic Markers were essential for her—and their effectiveness compares most favorably with expensive flannel board and charts used today." Dr. Roberts didn't pass up modern techniques, however. As time passed, she adopted slides and tapes. She collaborated on at least one instructional movie. She must have loved overhead projectors when they became available—though it is certain she would never have tolerated their use for pages of closely spaced typewritten material.

Perhaps some of Dr. Roberts's interest in the how-tos of teaching went back to her days in elementary-school classrooms. She believed in observation and in learning by doing as well as in learning by reading and writing. For example, she liked for students in her classes to actually weigh out 100-calorie portions of food, or the amount of broccoli or orange juice required to provide the daily allowance of vitamin C. From exercises such as these came a teaching aid that was widely used for many years. A student described its beginning:

> *Another example of Miss Roberts's fine teaching methods was the development of models of 100-calorie portions of common foods. The foods in 100-calorie portions were set up in a lab and an artist drew accurate and life size pictures of them. These drawings were printed on drawing paper and sold in tablet form. These then were colored in crayon, water color or oil by the user, then cut out and mounted on wooden blocks. They were a marvellous teaching device and so easy to carry round and set up for a class discussion or a PTA meeting.*

Similar models were later printed in full color on light-weight posterboard, die-cut so that they could easily be punched out. These were distributed by the National Dairy Council for many years.

Dr. Roberts also liked students to have the opportunity to observe nutrition programs in action. She had started this type of observation with the program in the Free Dispensary when she was a new faculty member at the University of Chicago. Through the years, other types of experience were added—observation in clinics, dietary departments, and the University of Chicago nursery school. "Part of the classroom work," one student wrote, "was to visit various child nutrition projects going on in the Chicago area. I recall visiting at least five such projects . . . I thought later that these could be considered an early form of clinical experience comparable to some in coordinated undergraduate programs."

As another form of learning involvement, Dr. Roberts thought it important for students to have some experience with research early in their graduate programs. When a research project was under way in the department, she sought, whenever it was feasible, to give students other than those directly responsible the opportunity to observe and participate. One student recounted:

> *I remember when the study was going on at the St. George School on Drexel*

Avenue. I acted as recorder for one of the pediatricians in the initial examination of the children. My most vivid memory, however, is of going to the school early *on some mornings when breakfast servings were to be weighed out! There were other activities, too, all of which were useful to me later when I was doing my own research. . . and then I, in turn, appreciated the help of fellow students.*

As in every graduate program, seminars played an important part in the educational process for Dr. Roberts's students. For those presenting the results of their research, the seminars provided an opportunity for using all they had learned about clear presentations and good visual aids. Because other students in the seminar had often had some part—even though small—in the work of the research project being presented, they listened with close attention and learned to question effectively. There was another fringe benefit associated with University of Chicago seminars, too, which a former student and staff member recalled:

Miss Roberts had a lot of friends among important nutritionists of the day, especially those like Dr. McCollum, Dr. Wilder and Dr. Tom Spies. . . whenever any of these people happened to be going through Chicago, they always seemed to call her, and she would get them to come out and give a . . . seminar to her graduate students. That helped us to feel that we knew who these people were whose publications and whose books we had been reading.

The seminars in Blaine Hall were always preceded by tea, and in that social period students often had a chance to really talk to those people who had only been names before.

As another form of student involvement, Dr. Roberts sometimes arranged for graduate students to attend meetings in which she was a participant. One person told of having attended a meeting of the Food and Nutrition Board committee working on the first revision of the Recommended Dietary Allowances—a committee that Dr. Roberts chaired. "We sat in a row along one wall of the room, taking it all in," she said. "We were amused when one of the men turned to Miss Roberts and asked, 'Who is the gallery?'"

Lydia Roberts was interested in nutrition education for people of all ages, of course, but she always had a special interest and involvement in programs directed toward children. She had a strong personal conviction, starting with her work in the Free Dispensary, that early nutrition education could help solve the problem of malnourished children. This strong interest, combined with her experience as an elementary teacher, gave her a special skill in presenting nutrition information to children—and children were one of her favorite audiences. Many students profited from the opportunity of watching her in action, and they commented on it in their letters. One person gave this example:

> *She gave vivid demonstrations of nutrition lessons suited to children. . . I remember her use of two test tubes of solution of an iron salt—one pale and one bright red—asking children to describe someone with blood of each type. She then tied these observations together with identification of all types of green vegetables as sources of iron. (We weren't so concerned about availability of iron in 1938 as we are now.) She had equally dramatic ways of teaching dietary sources of calcium and various vitamins of concern at the time.*

Although Dr. Roberts especially enjoyed working with children, she certainly did not limit her efforts to them. She believed in reaching as many people as possible through whatever means were feasible—articles in lay publications, talks, exhibits, demonstrations, skits. She felt that nutrition research achieved its greatest importance when it was translated into terms that ordinary people could understand and put into practice. As far as she was concerned, she could never overstress the importance of the practical application of nutrition knowledge, and she made her students feel this, too. "A concept I learned from her was that nutrition teaching should result in improved *practices*," one student wrote. Others commented on her ability "to put nutritional knowledge to practical application" or "to project the practical applications of ongoing research." One student said that "one of the most valuable things she taught me was to use common sense in handling nutrition problems."

This emphasis on practical application was always a distinguishing characteristic of Dr. Roberts's work. In her early years in nutrition she had stressed this interest in many articles she wrote for lay publications. During the time she was at the University of Chicago, she made an effort to reach teachers, public health workers, and others interested in nutrition through special summer courses that stressed practical application of nutrition knowledge.

These interesting and innovative courses, which were offered in addition to the regular class schedule, fully utilized the principles of demonstration, observation, and participation that Dr. Roberts thought important. The summer of 1940 was special, for it was the first time that Dr. Roberts offered one of her famous nutrition workshops, which later became a sort of trademark for her.

The basic technique of the workshop method is the use of the Socratic system of asking questions, defining problems, and developing answers. Although the method applies to many fields, it has proved to be particularly useful for instructing students and workers in practical nutrition. Participants bring their problems to the workshop and the group works out solutions under the guidance of the leader or leaders.

The first workshop, in 1940, was held in Dr. Roberts's home area of Allegan County, Michigan, and was sponsored by the W. K. Kellogg Foundation, the Michigan Department of Health, and the School Master's Club of Allegan. The workshop was a follow-up of a special program in child care and home hygiene for teachers of home economics or biology in Michigan high schools. The 1940 program was open to principals, teachers, nurses, and others responsible for the health and welfare of children. Its purpose was to study the health and nutrition problems of a community and the ways and means of coordinating its resources in dealing with those problems.[2]

After this successful start, workshops continued to be a feature of summer-session programs during the remainder of Dr. Roberts's time at the University of Chicago. A wide variety of topics were covered, with the ones in nutrition concentrating on problems of community nutrition, particularly as they related to the war and the national-defense effort. Although the leadership of these workshops was centered in the faculty of the Department of Home Economics, many outstanding speakers and leaders were made available through the cooperation of agencies such as the Children's Bureau, the Department of Labor, and the McCormick Memorial Fund.

One of the most exciting and effective workshops of the University of Chicago period was held in 1942. Earlier that year, Dr. Roberts had made a special tour to observe nutrition problems in the South at the request of M. L. Wilson of the National Nutrition Committee. Apparently, her observations on this tour influenced the choice of the general topic of the workshop, which was on low-income diets—what the diets of people in low-income areas were like, and how they could be improved in simple, practical ways. Of the 59 participants in the month-long workshop, 16 came from the South, some, undoubtedly, as the result of encounters on Dr. Roberts's tour. A list of participants prepared for the 1942 workshop by Dr. Roberts indicates that as far as she was concerned, the "participants" included all those involved in the workshop—faculty as well as students. A person who came in to give one lecture or to spend one session with the workshop was not listed as a participant, but all others were, because all were working together.

To define the problems for the 1942 workshop, diets of low-income families in various parts of the country were evaluated. Most of the diets considered were those of rural populations, but, since this was wartime, food intakes of some urban populations, particularly those of industrial workers, also were considered. With the problems identified, practical ways of dealing with them were discussed. A variety of teaching materials, such as skits and children's books, were prepared by workshop participants. These, along with readily available materials from government and commercial sources, were evaluated and discussed, as were different ways in which people could be encouraged to become involved and interested. The solutions proposed by the group involved more than just educational materials, however. Topics such as increasing the use of enriched flour or reaching workers in industrial plants also were considered, discussed, and later implemented by the participants.[3]

After Dr. Roberts left the University of Chicago, she continued to develop and refine the nutrition-workshop method in Puerto Rico. Eventually workshops were held throughout the Caribbean area. Sometimes the groups involved were very large. Some of the workshops had more than 150 participants, and were described by Dr. Roberts as "a three-ringed circus!" But no matter where workshops were held—in Chicago or in the Caribbean—or how large they became, they seemed to retain a quality of enthusiasm and spontaneity, reflecting, no doubt, the enthusiasm and spontaneity of Dr. Roberts herself, for she never seemed to "burn out." Indeed, one of the important factors in her success as a teacher appears to have been her contagious enthusiasm. It was not a legacy she could pass on to everyone, perhaps, but it could not help but influence many.

One former student offered this statement concerning Dr. Roberts's teaching. Most of her students would undoubtedly agree with the summary:

> *Dr. Roberts was a master teacher. She was not only knowledgeable about her field of expertise, but loved to impart her know-how to students. She did not stop with students, but seized every opportunity to spread the word about nutrition to anyone who could be influenced for the benefit of people—especially children.*

REFERENCES

1. Roberts LJ: Statement of Interests and Recent Activities of Lydia J. Roberts. Report on file. Chicago, University of Chicago Archives, 1938.
2. Dye M: *Home Economics at the University of Chicago, 1892–1956.* Chicago, University of Chicago Home Economics Alumni Association, 1972, p 82.
3. Dreis T: Report on workshop to M. L. Wilson, 1942. Washington, DC, personal files, Thelma Dreis.

CHAPTER 5

Appraise, Evaluate, Educate!

In research, as in teaching, Lydia Roberts was a strong advocate of practical application. In her view, the scientific facts learned in the laboratory should be applied to the practical problems of growth, development, and health maintenance. Scientific information on nutrition needs and processes should be combined with practical information on food, food habits, and food production. Social and psychological factors should be considered as well. Finally, it was of prime importance that the information should be communicated in an easily comprehended form. Because of these strongly held convictions, and her vigor in implementing them, few people have had greater influence in the field of applied nutrition than Dr. Roberts.

Dr. Roberts's interest in the practical, applied side of nutrition did not mean that she in any way belittled the importance of nutrition science—or that she was inadequate in conducting scientific research. Her own scientific training under Dr. Katharine Blunt and in the chemistry and physiology departments of the University of Chicago had been rigorous. She required the same for her students. Of the more than 100 publications listed in her bibliography, approximately a third appeared in scientific and professional journals of the highest caliber. Papers by her and her graduate students appeared in such publications as the *Journal of the American Medical Association*, the *Archives of Internal Medicine*, the *Journal of Pediatrics*, and the *American Journal of Diseases of Children*, as well as in the journals in which nutrition research more traditionally appears, such as the *Journal of Nutrition* and the *Journal of The American Dietetic Association.*

This impressive list of scientific publications was gratifying to Dr. Roberts, of course—but it represented only a part of what she worked to accomplish throughout her career. She wanted sound nutrition information, together with practical methods of applying that information, to reach the public. She never missed an opportunity to get nutrition information to people who needed it, and to get it to them in a form that they could use. As a result, an almost equal number of articles under her name appeared in publications for the lay public and for elementary- and secondary-school teachers. These papers bore such titles as "Teaching Children to Eat Good Breakfasts"[1] or "Cutting Down on Candy."[2] Most of the articles of this type appeared during her early years of teaching at the University of Chicago, before the administrative duties for the Department of Home Economics took up her time. She did not give up her interest in popular publications, however, and during her years in Puerto Rico, her name again appeared on publications such as *Mejor Arroz, Mejor Salud* (Better Rice, Better Health)[3] and *Alimentos Para Su Familia* (Food for Your Family).[4]

The remaining third of Dr. Roberts's publications appeared in a variety of forms—books, government bulletins, review articles, or interpretive articles in professional journals. They exemplified in various ways the three major areas of her professional interest and activity: nutrition investigation, nutrition education, and community nutrition.

With her belief that the ultimate goal of nutrition research was for human betterment, it is not surprising that virtually all of Dr. Roberts's research involved human subjects. Only one of her published papers, in fact, reported a research study on animals.[5] That paper, a report on the relation of liver stores of vitamin A to the early signs of deficiency of the vitamin in rats, was actually only one part of a larger study that did involve human subjects. One thing that never changed through Dr. Roberts's long professional life, whether in Michigan, Montana, Illinois, or Puerto Rico, was her interest in and love and concern for children. More than half of her publications, both those reporting on research and those intended for the lay public, dealt specifically with child nutrition.

In some of the ideas she presented in her papers, Dr. Roberts was ahead of her times. It was her conviction that nutritionists should not work in isolation, but should cooperate with workers in other disciplines. As early as 1924, she had expressed this idea in an article, "The Nutrition Specialist in the Health Program."[6] Other papers proposing or illustrating the value of the interdisciplinary approach followed: "The Place of Nutrition in the School Program,"[7] "The Psychologists Study Eating Habits,"[8] "The Dietitian in Social Service,"[9] and "The School Lunch as a Health Agency."[10] As Ethel Austin Martin pointed out in a review of Dr. Roberts's publications, "the concept of the nutritionist as a member of the health team is commonly accepted today. But more than forty years ago (1924) when Dr. Roberts wrote on the subject . . . it was a startling new idea, one which was to have implications for the future of nutrition service."[11]

In all of Dr. Roberts's research, the basic plan of action was essentially the same. The first step was assessment or appraisal. Actually, appraisal was the key to her approach to all kinds of problems and programs. Whether she was planning a research project, a university course of study, or a community-wide nutrition program, she first assessed the current situation and established a baseline. Her dedication to the principle of appraisal was well illustrated when she was asked to become head of the Department of Home Economics at the University of Puerto Rico. She stipulated in her acceptance that funds would be made available for a study of the current nutritional status of the people of Puerto Rico. The data gathered in this study were published in book form in 1949, as *Patterns of Living in Puerto Rican Families.*[12] It is evident from the title that, in Dr. Roberts's view, "assessment" and "appraisal" had come to include more than just food habits and nutritional status. In this approach she was also in the vanguard of the nutritionists who would come to look at many aspects of lifestyle in setting up nutrition programs.

With baseline data in hand from appraisal and assessment, and with problems identified, the next steps were to study the problems, to attempt to solve them, and to try to bring about change. Obviously, Dr. Roberts's methods and approaches varied, depending on the particular situation, but her aim was to favor the simple, practical approach whenever possible.

Evaluation was the final research step. What had been learned? What had been accomplished? Were the results significant? What factors affected the outcome? What further work needed to be done? In reading publications of the late 1920s and early 1930s, the modern researcher may well be envious of the amount of space available for the discussion of results. In today's world of the computer, elegant laboratory techniques, and sophisticated statistical analyses, some of these early studies seem cumbersome and outdated—but reading the detailed discussions reveals the basically sound nature of the research.

For Dr. Roberts, there always was one more question after the evaluation of the results—was there a practical application? Co-workers were impressed with her "ability and vigor in translating theory and plans into action programs. To her, nutritional knowledge was a stepping stone to application in such terms as food enrichment, school lunches for children, and home production programs."[11]

Toward the end of Dr. Roberts's career at the University of Chicago, in the years 1941 through 1945, she became well known for her service on the committee that developed the first set of Recommended Dietary Allowances. This was not a new interest for her, because essentially all of her research had been involved, directly or indirectly, with the problem of determining the requirements for various nutrients. A review of her publications shows the development of this interest.

Two of Dr. Roberts's early studies, done under the auspices of the Children's Bureau, were on the nutrient intake of children in Gary, Indiana,[13] and in a mountain county in Kentucky.[14] These were followed by studies on an Indian reservation[15] and of children in a preventorium.[16] Malnutrition was evident in all groups. Presumably the food intake of the children was inadequate in quality, quantity or both. How should the diets be modified? What kinds of food should be added or taken away? Few data were available to help answer the questions. Some help might be obtained by examining the differences between the diets of these children and those of children who were obviously well nourished. Following this logical progression, a series of detailed studies was carried out at the University of Chicago in the 1920s on the energy, protein, and mineral intake of well-nourished children.[17]

As the studies on appraisal of nutrient intakes progressed, inferences were drawn as to requirements for various nutrients. These led to further studies in the late 1930s and early 1940s aimed especially at studying the requirement for specific nutrients. Some of these projects were carried out as parts of larger dietary studies. Others took the form of detailed and lengthy balance studies. All involved the use of human subjects, and emphasis was placed on having the subjects lead lives as "normal" as possible—a challenge, no doubt, to the subjects as well as the investigators. As a result of these research projects, specific recommendations were made as to the requirements of children and adults for vitamins C and A and for iron; recommendations also were made concerning the requirements of young adults for riboflavin and thiamin.

Some of these studies on requirements became major research projects. A series of papers on vitamin A requirements was published between 1939 and 1942.[18–21] These involved both biochemical and dietary investigations, as well as extensive tests on the reliability of the adaptometer and the biophotometer as a means of measuring subclinical vitamin A deficiency. Vitamin C requirements of children of different ages were covered in another series of papers.[22–24] Studies on iron requirement fell into two categories, those involving young children[25] and those involving young women.[26,27] The latter studies, which followed the iron balances of a group of young women over a series of menstrual cycles, are regarded as classics for the detailed information they provided on the iron needs of women. Studies on the riboflavin and thiamin requirements of young women differed from most previously published studies in that they followed a group of subjects engaged in their usual student activities over a period of several months.[28,29]

All of this research was interesting and absorbing, but the studies in which Dr. Roberts seemed to have the most interest and most personal involvement were those having to do with children, particularly three major studies that dealt with the effect of specific dietary supplements. In 1938 Lydia Roberts made this statement:

> *It is my belief that the ultimate test of what constitutes an optimum diet must be made on human beings under normal conditions of living, and that a logical approach to this problem is through large scale feeding experiments in which the effect of adding basic foods to the diet is determined. If improvement does result, it indicates that the original diet was lacking in some of the dietary essentials supplied by the food.*[30]

This approach was followed in three major studies on children that were carried out under Dr. Roberts's direction in the late 1930s and early 1940s. The first of these studies examined the effect of adding a pint of milk to the diet of children in an institution.[31–33] The second involved the supplementation of what was considered to be a good diet with additional food—in this case, bananas.[34,35] In the third study, the results of providing a "liberally adequate" diet to children in a boarding school were evaluated.[36–38] As new techniques and new knowledge became available, there was an increase in the number of nutrients studied and measurements made. This was in line with Dr. Roberts's view that such studies should not supplant laboratory studies, but rather support and supplement them. In her opinion, the real advantage of such studies was that they afforded "the type of evidence that will be accepted by the lay public as showing that it does in reality make a difference whether a child receives a fully adequate diet or one giving only bare maintenance."[31] This was, no doubt, the kind of evidence she had been seeking as a teacher in Montana, and it was the kind she wanted the public to have.

Because these studies were of particular concern to Dr. Roberts, it is interesting to review them in terms of their contributions. The purpose of the first study was to determine whether adding a pint of milk to the diet of children already receiving about one pint of milk a day would result in any improvement in the children's physical condition. After an initial assessment period, children in the institution were divided into three groups of 36 children each. These groups were matched as equally as possible for age, sex, height, weight, and condition of teeth. One group served as a control, another group received a daily equivalent of one pint of milk in the form of evaporated milk, and the third received the same amount of irradiated evaporated milk. The supplements were continued for a full calendar year. The effect of the supplement was measured by growth in height and weight,[31] the rate of bone development as judged by x-ray films of the carpal bones,[32] and by the condition of the teeth at the beginning and end of the experimental year.[33] The results showed that by every method of measurement the children given either milk supplement fared better than children living on the regular institution diet.

In a supplementary study, measurements of capillary fragility, as determined by the Dalldorf resistometer, were carried out as an indication of the vitamin C status of the children.[22] The results indicated that the institution diet apparently was low in vitamin C except during the summer months, when tomatoes and vegetables were served fairly liberally. However, the validity of the measure of capillary fragility as an accurate indicator of vitamin C status was questioned. The results were probably disappointing in this respect, for the method had been suggested as a quick, easy, and inexpensive method of detecting subclinical vitamin C deficiency. Determinations of blood ascorbic acid levels were added in future studies.

The study on milk supplementation received widespread attention, and on the basis of this work, Dr. Roberts received the Borden Award in 1938. This award is given annually in recognition of outstanding research in nutrition. Dr. Roberts and the 1937 winner, Dr. Amy Daniels of the University of Iowa, were nominated by a committee of the American Home Economics Association. The awards—gold medals and checks for $1,000—were presented to Dr. Roberts and Dr. Daniels at the annual meeting of the association in 1938.

The second study on food supplementation was carried out in an institution for boys. In this case, the diet was considered to be fairly adequate in all nutrients, with the possible exception of vitamin C. The weight of most of the boys was in the "normal" range. One hundred of the boys received a dietary supplement of two to three bananas a day over the school year.[34] This involved, incidentally, over 48,000 bananas, an average of 459 per boy! Moreover, the bananas were well liked throughout the study and were, in fact, "eaten with the same relish and dispatch" at the end of the experiment as at the beginning.

The progress of the boys on the banana-supplemented diet was compared with a control group in the same institution. In addition to height, weight, and ossification of the carpals, Franzen indices also were determined.[34] In determining this index, an extensive set of body measurements is carried out that attempts to assess the relationship between the amount of soft tissue and the size of the skeleton. Measurements of capillary fragility and blood ascorbic acid levels also were made.[35]

The boys receiving the supplement showed consistently better growth and development than the controls, by every measure of physical status that was used. The authors pointed out that the differences were not statistically significant in most cases, but the fact that the observations were made on matched groups and were consistent in direction lent support to the belief that the differences were due to the supplement. The increase in the level of blood ascorbic acid was significant, however. The conclusion was that "these results indicate that the allowances for the various dietary essentials for boys of the age here studied should approach the higher rather than the minimum standards which have heretofore been proposed, in particular for vitamin C."[35]

The last of these large-scale studies on child nutrition was carried out shortly before Dr. Roberts's retirement from the University of Chicago. The subjects were students in a boarding school near the university, and included children in all the elementary grades. After a preliminary two-month period of appraisal and observation, the diet—which was considered to be "about average"—was supplemented by a number of foods (dairy products, eggs, whole-grain cereal and bread, and pineapple juice) to make it "liberally adequate." Results were judged by acceptance of the foods by the children, by changes in the nutritive value of the diet actually consumed, by growth in height and weight before, during, and after supplementation, and by changes in the nutritional status for thiamin, riboflavin, vitamin C, vitamin A, protein, and iron, as judged by appropriate blood or urinary studies.

The diet was well accepted by the children.[36] There appeared to be some improvement in the growth rate, although the results were not statistically significant.[37] Dietary analysis of the unsupplemented diet had indicated that the only undesirably low values were those for vitamin C and for thiamin. Plasma ascorbic acid and blood thiamin levels, which were low at the beginning of the study in many of the children, were significantly improved by the changes in the diet. Test dose returns and one-hour fasting excretions of thiamin also were improved. Riboflavin test dose returns, which were relatively high on the institutional diet, showed no significant change on the supplemented diet. Fasting one-hour excretions of riboflavin, however, were considerably higher in the spring than in the autumn. Altogether, the results of the biochemical studies were "in complete agreement" with those of the dietary studies. "This offers further support," the authors stated, "for the acceptance of biochemical measurements of nutritional status."[38]

As these studies on dietary supplementation in children developed over the years, they increased in sophistication and scope and contributed considerable evidence concerning the nutrient requirements of children of different ages. It seems safe to assume, however, that for Dr. Roberts, one of the main accomplishments of these studies was that they demonstrated that "diet makes a difference."

With her retirement from the University of Chicago in 1944 and her move to Puerto Rico, Dr. Roberts's involvement in laboratory-oriented nutrition research ended, although her data-gathering days certainly did not. Nor did her interest in the application of new nutrition knowledge come to an end—indeed, it might be said that she simply exchanged the scientific laboratories of the university for the laboratory of the community. Her techniques of bringing about dietary change were enlarged to include lobbying in the legislature, influencing advertisers, and selling government officials on the importance of better diets for better health. Certainly, in her new setting, Lydia Roberts found an unprecedented opportunity to be effective in her ultimate goal—to devote her efforts "to the problem of interpreting nutrition in terms of human requirements and to devising ways and means by which the nutrition knowledge we now have may be used for human betterment."[30]

REFERENCES

1. Roberts LJ: Teaching children to eat good breakfasts. *Normal Instructor and Primary Plans,* February 1931, p 70.
2. Roberts LJ: Cutting down on candy. *Hygeia* 2:411, 1924.
3. Roberts LJ: *Mejor Arroz, Mejor Salud.* San Juan, Puerto Rico Dept of Instruction, 1951.
4. Roberts LJ: *Alimentos Para Su Familia.* San Juan, Puerto Rico Dept of Instruction, 1952.
5. Brenner S, Brookes MCH, Roberts LJ: The relation of liver stores to the occurrence of early signs of vitamin A deficiency in the white rat. *J Nutr* 23:459, 1942.
6. Roberts LJ: The nutrition specialist in the health program. *Hosp Soc Ser* 9:245, 1924.
7. Roberts LJ: The place of nutrition in the school program. *Commonwealth* 15:77, 1928.
8. Roberts LJ: The psychologists study eating habits. *Child Study* 7:35, 1929.
9. Roberts LJ: The dietitian in social service. *J Am Diet Assoc* 5:286, 1930.
10. Roberts LJ: The school lunch as a health agency. *Hygeia* 12:753, 1934.
11. Martin EA: The life works of Lydia J. Roberts. *J Am Diet Assoc* 49:299, 1966.
12. Roberts LJ, Stefani RL: *Patterns of Living in Puerto Rican Families.* Río Piedras, PR, University of Puerto Rico, 1949.
13. Roberts LJ: *Children of Preschool Age in Gary, Indiana. II Diet of the Children.* Pub. no. 122. Washington, DC, US Children's Bureau, 1922.
14. Roberts LJ: *Diet and Care of Children in a Mountain County of Kentucky.* Pub. no. 110. Washington, DC, US Children's Bureau, 1922.
15. Stene JA, Roberts LJ: A nutrition study on an Indian reservation. *J Am Diet Assoc* 3:215, 1928.
16. Hord N, Roberts LJ: Results of dietary and hygienic control of ten non-gaining preventorium children. *J Am Diet Assoc* 4:77, 1928.
17. Wait B, Roberts LJ: Studies in the food requirement of adolescent girls. 1. The energy intake of well-nourished girls 10–16 years of age. 2. Daily variations in the energy intake of the individual. 3. The protein intake of well-nourished girls 10–16 years of age. 4. The mineral intake of 38 well-nourished girls 10–16 years of age. *J Am Diet Assoc* 8:209, 323, 1932; 8:403, 9:124, 1933.
18. Steininger G, Roberts LJ, Brenner S: Vitamin A in the blood of normal adults. The effect of a depletion diet on blood values and biophotometer readings. *JAMA* 113:2381, 1939.
19. Steininger G, Roberts LJ: Biophotometer test as an index of nutritional status for vitamin A. *Arch Intern Med* 64:1110, 1939.
20. Oldham HG, Roberts LJ, MacLennan K, Schultz FW: Dark adaptation of children in relation to dietary levels of vitamin A. *J Pediatr* 20:740, 1942.

21. Brenner S, Roberts LJ: Effects of vitamin A depletion in young adults. *Arch Intern Med* 71:474, 1943.
22. Roberts LJ, Blair R, Bailey M: Seasonal variations in capillary resistance of institution children. *J Pediatr* 11:626, 1937.
23. Roberts VM, Roberts LJ: A study of the ascorbic acid requirements of children of early school age. *J Nutr* 24:25, 1942.
24. Roberts VM, Brookes MH, Roberts LJ, Koch P, Shelby P: The ascorbic acid requirement of school age girls. *J Nutr* 26:539, 1943.
25. Johnston FA, Roberts LJ: The iron requirement of children of early school age. *J Nutr* 23:181, 1942.
26. Leverton RM, Roberts LJ: Hemoglobin and red cell content of the blood of normal women during successive menstrual cycles. *JAMA* 106:1459, 1936.
27. Leverton RM, Roberts LJ: The iron metabolism of normal young women during consecutive menstrual cycles. *J Nutr* 13:65, 1937.
28. Davis MV, Oldham HG, Roberts LJ: Riboflavin excretion of young women on diets containing varying levels of the B vitamins. *J Nutr* 32:143, 1946.
29. Oldham HG, Davis MV, Roberts LJ: Thiamin excretion and blood levels of young women on diets containing varying levels of the B vitamins, with some observations on niacin and pantothenic acid. *J Nutr* 32:163, 1946.
30. Roberts LJ: The Interests and Activities of Lydia J. Roberts. Report on file. Chicago, University of Chicago Archives, 1938.
31. Roberts LJ, Blair R, Lenning B, Scott M: Effect of a milk supplement on the physical status of institutional children. 1. Growth in height and weight. *Am J Dis Child* 56:287, 1938.
32. MacNair V, Roberts LJ: Effect of a milk supplement on the physical status of institutional children. 2. Ossification of the bones of the wrist. *Am J Dis Child* 56:494, 1938.
33. Roberts LJ, Engelbrecht S, Blair R, Williams W, Scott M: Effect of a milk supplement on the physical status of institutional children. 3. Progress of dental caries. *Am J Dis Child* 56:805, 1938.
34. Roberts LJ, Blair R, Austin G, Steininger G: The supplementary value of the banana in institution diets. 1. Effect on growth in height and weight, ossification of carpals, and changes in Franzen indices. *J Pediatr* 15:25, 1939.
35. Roberts LJ, Brookes MH, Blair R, Austin G, Noble I: The supplementary value of banana in institution diets. 2. Capillary resistance and reduced ascorbic acid in the blood plasma. *J Pediatr* 15:43, 1939.
36. Roberts LJ, Blair R, Greider M: Results of providing a liberally adequate diet to children in an institution. 1. Acceptance of foods and adequacy of diets consumed. *J Pediatr* 27:393, 1945.
37. Blair R, Roberts LJ, Greider M: Results of providing a liberally adequate diet to children in an institution. 2. Growth in height and weight. *J Pediatr* 27:410, 1945.
38. Oldham HG, Roberts LJ, Young M: Results of providing a liberally adequate diet to children in an institution. 3. Blood and urinary excretion studies before and after dietary improvement. *J Pediatr* 27:418, 1945.

CHAPTER 6

Outside the Halls of Ivy

Lydia Roberts was not a person who would have been satisfied to spend all her time in the "halls of ivy," no matter how satisfying the work in the laboratory or classroom might be. In her view, ensuring the practical application of sound nutrition principles required personal involvement in the decision-making process, whether it be at the local, national or international level. That meant going outside the university.

This type of involvement had been stressed in the Department of Home Economics of the University of Chicago since its early days. In a 1925 report on the work of the department, Dr. Katharine Blunt dealt at some length with the topic of "the Department's contribution to community and national welfare."[1] Dr. Roberts had played an active role in such activities at that time. She increased her involvement as time passed, even after she had assumed added administrative duties as head of the department.

As the years passed, Lydia Roberts became a familiar figure in the conference rooms where important national committees debated nutrition-related problems. Her book on child nutrition, her research publications, and her popular articles on nutrition were supplemented by addresses and talks to both professional and lay groups. As she herself described her broad range of activities, she had "given talks on subjects in line with my general field of interest before numerous groups who are in a position to influence the nutrition of children, such as Home Economics teachers, dietitians, dentists, public health offices, workers in child development, parents, and other scientific and lay groups, and have written numerous articles on similar topics for scientific and popular journals."[2]

Much of Dr. Roberts's activity in the field of public service centered in Chicago, where she held such assignments as chairman of the Budget Committee for the Chicago Council of Social Agencies, chairman of the Chicago Nutrition Council, and member of the Council on Food and Nutrition of the American Medical

Association. As the years passed, her activities broadened. More and more often, her sister Lillian packed Lydia's suitcase for professional trips to all parts of the country. More and more frequently, especially during World War II, these trips were to Washington, DC—and finally to Puerto Rico. Such activities established her as a molder of nutrition policy and made her a figure of national importance in the nutrition field.

Lydia Roberts's involvement in public service started early in her second career and was no doubt encouraged by the "nutrition environment" at the time of her entry into the field. In 1918, when she finished her master's degree and became a member of the University of Chicago faculty, wartime interest in nutrition was high. Interest in child health and nutrition was increasing. Under the auspices of the Children's Bureau, a Children's Year was declared in 1918. A bulletin, *What Is Malnutrition?,* written by Lydia Roberts, was one of a series of Children's Bureau publications that came about as a result of the Children's Year. The bulletin outlined and discussed what was known at the time about the causes, effects, and treatment of malnutrition in children. It was revised and republished by the bureau in 1927.[3]

During the period following the Children's Year, in the early 1920s, the Children's Bureau actively encouraged research in the field of child nutrition. Lydia Roberts's studies in Gary, Indiana, and in a mountain county in Kentucky were carried out for the bureau.[4,5] Even before the final reports on these studies were published in 1922, however, her activities in the field of child nutrition had led to other important assignments.

In 1921, Lydia Roberts was appointed to the Child Health Council's National Advisory Committee on Foods and Nutrition. Of the 27 members of the committee, 12 represented national organizations interested in nutrition, such as the Department of Agriculture, the American Red Cross, and the American Home Economics Association. The remaining members of the committee were selected because of their expertise in the field of child nutrition. The committee was formed "in order that the Council might secure a consensus of authoritative opinion regarding policies, methods and standards which are essential to the effective conduct of nutrition work."[6]

The names of the members of this group read like a nutrition who's who. Among the 27 members were J. R. Murlin, Graham Lusk, Henry C. Sherman, Lafayette B. Mendel, Joseph Goldberger, E. V. McCollum, W. P. R. Emerson, Mary Swartz Rose, Amy Daniels, Agnes Fay Morgan, and Lucy Gillett. Other members were distinguished, too, but these had already made their mark in nutrition or were soon to do so. Many of them were Lydia Roberts's contemporaries, but they had already been at work in the field of nutrition for some time. Indeed, to be appointed to this committee must have been quite a feather in the cap of a woman who had received her master's degree only three years earlier, who had been in the academic world for only four years, and whose publications were still limited. Apparently those appointing the committee could recognize ability when they saw it, even in its early stages.

It seems likely that service on this committee provided Lydia Roberts with her first opportunity to become personally acquainted with some of these people. They came from different parts of the country and represented a number of disciplines. Some were biochemists, some were clinicians, some were in research, and some were in administrative positions of various sorts. All were united in their common interest in nutrition. Lydia Roberts established close friendships with many of her co-workers on this and subsequent assignments—friendships that lasted for many years, and that were productive both personally and professionally.

Her work on the Children's Bureau projects and on the Child Health Council's committee ushered in what must have been an exciting decade, professionally, for Lydia Roberts. During the 1920s she completed the work for her doctorate, published her book, *Nutrition Work With Children*, and established the reputation for teaching and research that would lead to her appointment as head of the Home Economics Department at the University of Chicago. It was also a period in which research in nutrition was producing an extraordinary influx of new and exciting knowledge. Interest in using this new knowledge for human betterment was high, and interest in child welfare, including child nutrition, was receiving much attention. The high point of this activity came in July 1929, when President Herbert Hoover issued a call for a White House Conference on Child Health and Protection. Lydia Roberts was an active participant in the conference, serving on three committees and chairing one dealing with nutrition service in schools.

This conference was the third White House Conference on children. The first, called by President Theodore Roosevelt in 1909, was concerned with dependent children. The stimulus of this conference led to the formation of the Children's Bureau in 1912. The second was called by President Woodrow Wilson in 1919 as the closing activity of the Children's Year of 1918. Both of these conferences were relatively small—about 200 delegates were present at each one. The scope of the second conference was enlarged, however, by a series of regional conferences.[7]

The 1930 conference was on a much larger scale. Some 3,000 men and women, leaders in the medical, educational, and social fields as they touched the lives of children, were in attendance at the meeting, held in Washington on 19 through 22 November 1930. Sixteen months of preparation, research, and study by nearly 1,200 experts working on 150 committees had gone into the presentation of the material. From Dr. Roberts's committee had come strong recommendations that nutrition teaching should be included in health-education programs for all children, both boys and girls, in every school grade. It was further stressed that the subject matter taught should be scientifically sound and suited to the age, intelligence, and interest of the children, with emphasis on the positive effects of good nutrition, rather than the bad effects of poor food habits.[7]

As a former elementary-school teacher, Dr. Roberts believed that the public school was the agency that should be looked to for the most widespread and effective nutrition education. This was one area, however, in which she was not able to see much progress. Even though there were many specific examples, such as those provided by her own research studies, where nutrition education and changes had brought about marked improvement in the health of children, there was not a widespread adoption of nutrition-education programs in school. Dr. Roberts summed it up in a 1940 article: ". . . For the country as a whole, this would appear to be still largely a neglected field. . . . It must be admitted . . . that in the rank and file of schools, little effective nutrition work has been accomplished. This is due primarily to the fact that nutrition is a specialized field, and the training of the teachers has neither made them aware of the problem nor prepared them to handle it."[8] However, Lydia Roberts was not discouraged easily. There had been progress, she thought, "although it is small when measured against the need that still exists." Even small progress was sufficient for her to continue to fight.

In the 1930s, Dr. Roberts's new responsibilities as head of the Department of Home Economics undoubtedly took up much of her time. Even so, she was still involved in other activities in addition to teaching and research. In 1934, she became a member of the Committee on Food and Nutrition of the American Medical Association. She served with this group—which soon became known as the American Medical Association Council on Food and Nutrition—until 1948, when she resigned because of her increasing activities in Puerto Rico.

The years that Dr. Roberts served on this council were important ones in terms of nutrition. In 1934, when she first became a member, the country was just beginning to emerge from the depression. A few years later, World War II brought new problems. Even before the United States entered the war, nutritionists were concerned with problems of supplying sufficient nutrients for people at home, of shipping food overseas, of feeding the army—the list was long. Enriching and fortifying foods to provide the highest return on the nutrition dollar was an important development of those years. Although *nutrition policy* was not a catchword of the times, as it became later, the Council on Foods and Nutrition was essentially making recommendations that influenced food and agriculture policies for the country.

For Dr. Roberts, the chance to work on such problems must have been challenging—a golden opportunity for practical application and utilization of nutrition knowledge. Again she had the privilege of working with outstanding people. Because of the council's association with the American Medical Association, many of its members were clinicians, but biochemists and nutritionists were included also. Dr. Roberts and the one other woman member of the council, Dr. Mary Swartz Rose of Columbia University, had important roles to play. Dr. Franklin Bing, who was the secretary of the Committee on Foods and Nutrition when Dr. Roberts was appointed, has told how for many years these women were depended on to present the views of nutritionists in council deliberations. Dr. Roberts's service often was sought between the council meetings as well. Dr. Ruth Cowan Clouse, who had received her doctorate in nutrition under Dr. Katharine Blunt's direction, was a member of the council staff—and also a close friend of Dr. Roberts. Dr. Bing has recounted how Dr. Clouse often took questions directly to Dr. Roberts

> *. . . over the weekends, for example, when she would be a guest at the cottage in the Indiana Dunes. . . . When on Mondays Dr. Clouse would come into the office, she would have with her a well thought-out plan for the consideration of the Council as a whole, on matters such as strained meats in the diets of infants, what the Council policy should be toward commercial diets for young children, or perhaps, how the nutritive value of certain foods might be properly described in advertising.*[9]

During Dr. Roberts's term of service, the council studied and made recommendations on topics such as the cereal-enrichment program, iodinization of salt, and fortification of milk with vitamin D. Council members also considered such problems as the necessity of restraining overzealous manufacturers in the vitamin supplementation of foods. Monitoring advertising and nutrition claims for products was another important activity. The council prepared and published a widely used *Handbook of Nutrition* during this period.[10] Dealing with such practical problems must have been of real interest to Dr. Roberts. What better way could there be to "spread the nutrition gospel," especially among clinicians?

In 1940 Dr. Roberts assumed another task, which was destined to become one of her most important activities. In that year, with Europe already at war and war clouds gathering for the United States in both the East and the West, the federal government requested that a committee on food and nutrition be set up under the National Research Council of the National Academy of Sciences.

The committee was formed, and, in 1941, it was set up on a permanent basis as the Food and Nutrition Board.

The leading nutritionists of that time were the obvious choice for membership on this important committee. For various reasons a policy had been established of not asking anyone over 60 to serve as a member. Unfortunately, this eliminated some outstanding people. E. V. McCollum, Henry Sherman, John R. Murlin, and Mary Swartz Rose were all ineligible. And, according to this criterion, so should Dr. Roberts have been. She was 61 in June 1940, but no one knew her age. In line with her usual practice, her birth year was not listed in *American Men of Science,* nor in any of the other commonly available sources of such information. It is possible that those setting up the committee did not check on Dr. Roberts very carefully, for certainly her level of vigor and activity belied her years. They may not have realized that she was nearly 40 when she entered the nutrition field. At any rate, Dr. Roberts was asked to join the board. She was not an illegal member for long, however. The policy on age was soon changed, and all of the "oldsters," except Mary Swartz Rose, who was ill, served on the committee during the next few years.[9]

It was the board's good fortune that Dr. Roberts was a member of the first group, for it was under her direction that one of the major accomplishments of the Food and Nutrition Board came about. The board recognized that one of its first functions should be to recommend the amounts of various nutrients that should be provided for the armed forces and also for the general population. Before this could be done, however, some sort of standards needed to be established.

Efforts had been made in the past, of course, to establish criteria for the requirements for various nutrients. Henry C. Sherman had set standards for adults for protein, calcium, phosphorus, and iron. Lucy Gillett had worked out calorie standards for children. The Technical Committee on Nutrition of the League of Nations, under the leadership of Dr. Mary S. Rose, had proposed standards for some nutrients. Dr. Hazel Stiebeling had proposed a set of standards for use by the US Department of Agriculture. But, as Dr. Roberts pointed out, "the existing standards were not only few but conflicting, and there were none that covered all nutrients for all ages and conditions."[11] Some sort of "nutrition yardstick" obviously was needed, but apparently even this committee of experts was unaware of the problems involved in developing such a guide. Dr. Roberts has given a much-quoted account of the dilemma:

> *How little the size of this problem was realized is shown by the fact that at the close of one day's meeting, Dr. Wilder appointed a committee of three—Dr. Helen Mitchell, Dr. Hazel Stiebeling and myself—to prepare a*

set of standards during the evening and be ready to present them to the group the next morning! We three spent the evening threshing over the problem (while the men, we felt sure, were out seeing the town). The result was, of course, that the only report we could bring in the next morning was that it couldn't be done, that the evidence was too scanty and too conflicting.[11]

Other members of the board didn't completely agree with Dr. Roberts's description. Dr. Bing came to their defense:

Miss Roberts was joking when she said that. She knew that Dr. Wilder had assignments for everyone, and that he often continued meetings after dinner, and called them for Saturday afternoons and all day Sundays, if need be, in those days. Nor does she tell the whole story. She did report promptly, as requested, and she did furnish figures for about ten important nutrients, including calories, to serve as a rough guide for immediate use. At the same time she emphasized the importance of the assignment, and expressed the desire that it be handled in a manner that would produce figures which the experts who might use them would be willing to accept. . . . It was under these conditions that a committee on dietary allowances was established, with a very sprightly 61-year-old as its chairman.[9]

With Dr. Roberts at the helm, it was not surprising that the committee started its work with a complete review of all the research reports in the literature that threw any light on the requirements for any of the nutrients under consideration. Even in today's world of computer searches of the literature, it would be a big job—at that time it must have seemed monumental. Each committee member took responsibility for certain nutrients, and probably instituted much the same system that Dr. Roberts put to work in Chicago. Everybody was involved—graduate students, faculty members, class participants—and all contributed to the search.

When all the information had been gathered—and the task was accomplished in a surprisingly short time—the committee formulated a tentative set of values for the various nutrients and conditions. These tentative figures were sent to a group of more than 50 nutritionists, because, as Dr. Roberts explained, the committee "believed that any accepted allowances should represent not just the thought of a small group of workers, however competent they might be, but that all persons who had done research on any factor or who had other bases for judgment should have a part in their formulation."[11] The response was excellent. Most of the 50 workers took time to reply and to give their judgments about the requirement for one or more of the nutrients, together with the evidence on which they based their comments.

The democratic process was continued with the next step. The suggestions received were studied, tabulated, evaluated, and, as far as possible, reconciled. A revised set of allowances was prepared and sent to the contributors, together with a summary of all the suggestions that had been received for each nutrient. Again, comments were requested, received, and a few additional revisions were made to harmonize all the suggestions as well as possible. In her article on the beginning of the Recommended Dietary Allowances (RDAs), Dr. Roberts did not really indicate how much work was involved in carrying out this review process. A folder of correspondence dating back to this period is among Dr. Roberts's papers in the Sala Roberts (Roberts Room) at the University of Puerto Rico. In it are some of the often-lengthy communications that were received by the committee. In every case, Dr. Roberts had written a considered, thoughtful reply, often telling in some detail the reasoning behind the committee's decision as to what the RDA for a given nutrient should be.[12]

The final test of the committee's work came with the presentation of the proposed RDAs to the members of the American Institute of Nutrition at their annual meeting in 1941. Dr. Roberts has described the presentation:

> *The wide interest in the problem was evidenced by the fact that the room was packed. It was with some trepidation that I, as chairman of the Committee, faced that group of distinguished research workers to present the allowances. We fully expected criticism and disagreement, if not attack, on their validity. I remember that as I sat in front of the room waiting for the audience to assemble Dr. Tom Spies, who was a member of the Board and sensed my feeling, stepped quietly up and whispered, "Remember, you are among friends!"*
>
> *There were questions and some comments, but to our surprise, no serious disagreements or attack. Why? For one reason, many of those present had already had their say in the matter. Others who might have held different opinions had no evidence to support them and being scientists would not speak until they had.*[11]

With the acceptance of the RDAs by the American Institute of Nutrition—"for the time being, at least," as Dr. Roberts said—the next step was presenting them to the National Nutrition Conference for Defense held in Washington on 26 through 28 May 1941.

Again, it was Dr. Roberts who presented the proposed RDAs at this conference. In line with her usual practical approach, she made sure that her audience, which included physicians, social workers, labor representatives, economists, food manufacturers, and others as well as nutritionists, understood just what these allowances would mean in terms of everyday food. A report in the *Journal of the Amer-*

ican Medical Association published shortly after the conference quoted her presentation:

> *The recommended allowances for food which this committee has agreed on are expressed in laboratory terms. Here is a daily diet which would measure up to these proposals: One pint of milk for an adult and more for a child; a serving of meat, and cheaper cuts are just as nutritious; one egg or some suitable substitute, such as navy beans; two vegetables, one of which should be green or yellow; two fruits, one of which should be rich in vitamin C, found abundantly in citrus fruit and tomatoes; breads, flour and cereal, most or preferably all whole grain or enriched; some butter or oleomargarine with vitamin A added; other foods to satisfy the appetite.*[13]

The first edition of the RDAs appeared in typescript, but it was published in the *Journal of The American Dietetic Association* within a couple of months.[14] It was not until 1943 that the official printed version appeared.[15] By this time it was already widely used. Obviously the RDAs had fulfilled a long-felt need.

In presenting the proposed allowances, the Food and Nutrition Board had stressed the fact that they were allowances, not requirements, and that they were based on the best knowledge available at the time. As more evidence became available, they would be subject to change.

Dr. Roberts was still chairman of the committee when the first revision of the RDAs was undertaken in 1944. Again, the democratic process was much in evidence, with 25 people meeting to discuss the issues. In Dr. Roberts's folder of correspondence concerning the revision of the RDAs, there was a statement she had prepared as opening remarks for this meeting. There had been considerable discussion, apparently, as to what level of adequacy the allowances should represent. In her remarks, she had this comment:

> *The level aimed at was not one on which individuals can "get by" without showing outward signs of deficiency, nor one clearly above any possible need. What we hoped to attain was the level of "comfort," one which provides enough for every organ and tissue for its best health and functioning.*[12]

She went on to discuss what she considered to be the responsibility of the committee in setting up the standards:

> *I need not emphasize the importance of this decision. The Dietary Allowances. . . are the official standards for the Quartermaster's office on feeding the armed forces; they are the guide in government plans and publications and are used in all civilian programs. It is our obligation, therefore, to be sure that the values are safe, but not extravagant. If our riboflavin and thiamin values, for example, are over generous, it puts an*

unnecessary burden on all these groups in trying to attain them, and constitutes an economic waste. On the other hand, if we set them too low for long continued use, we may be responsible for endangering the health of the armed forces and the civilian population. I think we would all agree that if anything we should err on the side of generosity rather than niggardliness, but that we do not want our values to be definitely in excess of any possible needs if we can decide what the level should be.[12]

Significant changes in the recommended allowances for riboflavin and thiamin were made at the time of the 1944 revision. Since the publication of the first revision in 1945, the RDAs have been reviewed and revised at about five-year intervals. They have served as guidelines for dietary evaluation in many nutrition studies. An important function has been their role as a unifying factor—a common ground for comparing different projects. In the view of Dr. Roberts, however, "one of the greatest services they have rendered has been to stimulate research to determine requirements for the various nutrients. The review of evidence by the Committee had revealed great gaps in our knowledge, and workers were challenged to fill in those gaps."[11]

In addition to Dr. Roberts's work on the development of the RDAs, for which she received the greatest recognition, she also served on the Food and Nutrition Board's Executive Committee, the Committee on Puerto Rican Nutrition, the Committee on Milk, the Committee on Nutrition of Industrial Workers, and the Committee on the Nutritional Aspect of Aging.[17] During her years of service on the board, 1940 through 1948, World War II and its aftermath forced the growth and use of nutrition knowledge, both for the armed services and for rehabilitating the populations of war-devastated countries. Lydia Roberts could not have found a better way in which to make practical application of nutrition knowledge.

Indirectly, Lydia Roberts's work on the Food and Nutrition Board led to another type of nutrition service and, ultimately, to her third career. She was in Washington, DC, for one of the board meetings in 1942 when M. L. Wilson, chairman of the National Nutrition Committee, approached her concerning a nutrition problem in Puerto Rico. During the years in which it had been a US Territory, the island of Puerto Rico had imported much of its food. Now, with wartime curtailment and diversion of shipping, food supplies were not reaching the island in the customary amounts. At the same time, the need for food had increased, since American troops were stationed on the island. Mr. Wilson asked Dr. Roberts if, on an upcoming visit to Puerto Rico, she would be willing to survey the nutrition situation and give him her thoughts on how the Nutrition Committee might be helpful on the island. The trip was made during her free quarter from the university in the winter of 1943. Her stay in Puerto Rico at that time was only six weeks long, but the die had been cast. The food and nutrition problems of Puerto Rico would concern Lydia Roberts for the rest of her life.

REFERENCES

1. Dye M: *Home Economics at the University of Chicago, 1892–1956.* Chicago, University of Chicago Home Economics Alumni Association, 1972, p 61.
2. Roberts LJ: Statement of Interests and Recent Activities of Lydia Roberts. Report on file. Chicago, University of Chicago Archives, 1938.
3. Roberts LJ: *What Is Malnutrition?* Pub. no. 59. Washington, DC, US Children's Bureau, 1917, revised 1927.
4. Roberts LJ: *The Nutrition and Care of Children in a Mountain County in Kentucky.* Pub. no. 110. Washington, DC, US Children's Bureau, 1922.
5. Roberts LJ: *Children of Pre-School Age in Gary, Indiana. II. Diet of the Children.* Pub. no. 122. Washington, DC, US Children's Bureau, 1922.
6. Notes from the field. *J Home Econ* 13:381, 1921.
7. *White House Conference, 1930, Addresses and Abstracts of Committee Reports.* New York, Century, 1931, p 176.
8. Roberts LJ: Status of nutrition work with children. *Ann Am Acad Pol Soc Sci* November 1940, p 111.
9. Bing FJ: Lydia J. Roberts—a biographical sketch. *J Nutr* 93:1, 1967.
10. Council on Food and Nutrition: *Handbook of Nutrition.* Chicago, American Medical Association, 1943.
11. Roberts LJ: Beginnings of the recommended dietary allowances. *J Am Diet Assoc* 34:903, 1958.
12. Correspondence on Recommended Dietary Allowances. Sala Roberts, School of Home Economics, University of Puerto Rico, Río Piedras.
13. Editorial, National Nutrition Congress for Defense. *JAMA* 116:2598, 1941.
14. The American Dietetic Association: Recommended allowances for the various dietary essentials. *J Am Diet Assoc* 17:565, 1941.
15. National Research Council: *Recommended Dietary Allowances.* Reprint and circular series no. 115. Washington, DC, National Research Council, 1943.
16. *The Food and Nutrition Board, 1940–65—Twenty-five Years in Retrospect.* Washington, DC, National Research Council, 1945.
17. *Proceedings,* vol 25. Washington, DC, National Research Council, 1965, p 33.

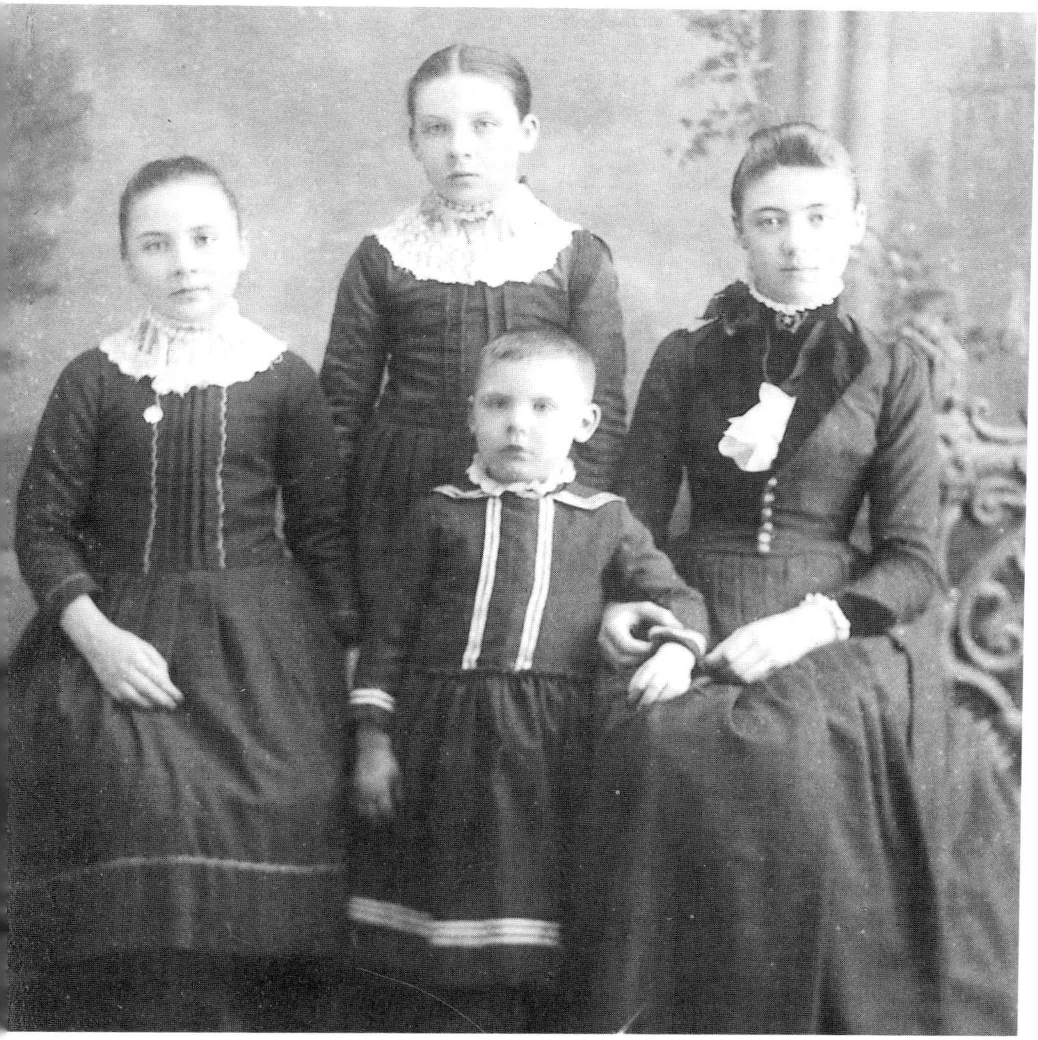

The Roberts family. John (front), surrounded by Lillian (left), Lydia (center), and Mary ("Mame," right). Photo by W.H. Blair, courtesy Hazel O'Connor.

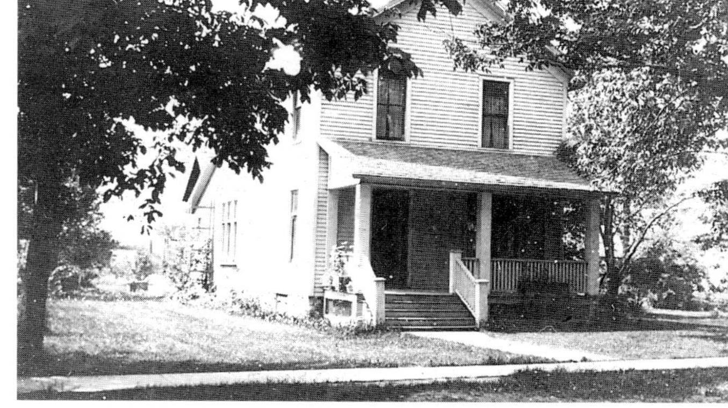

The Roberts home on Allegan Street, Martin, Michigan.

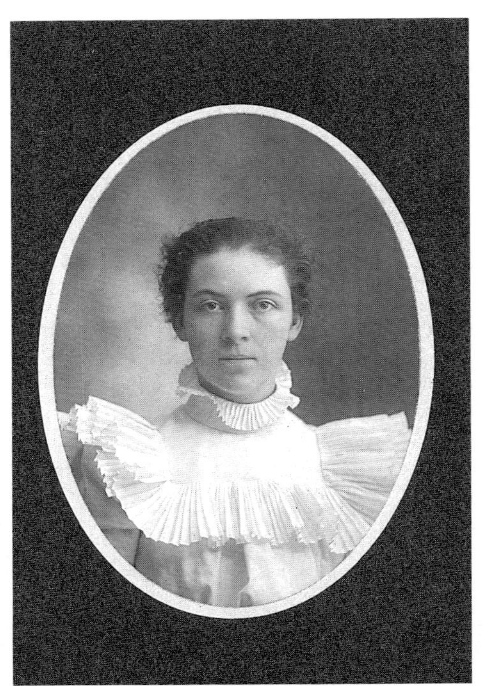

Lydia Roberts at about age 20, when she received a Limited Certificate from the Normal School, Mount Pleasant, Michigan. Photo courtesy Hazel O'Connor.

At work in her office in Blaine Hall at the University of Chicago, 1935. Photo by Ruth Blair.

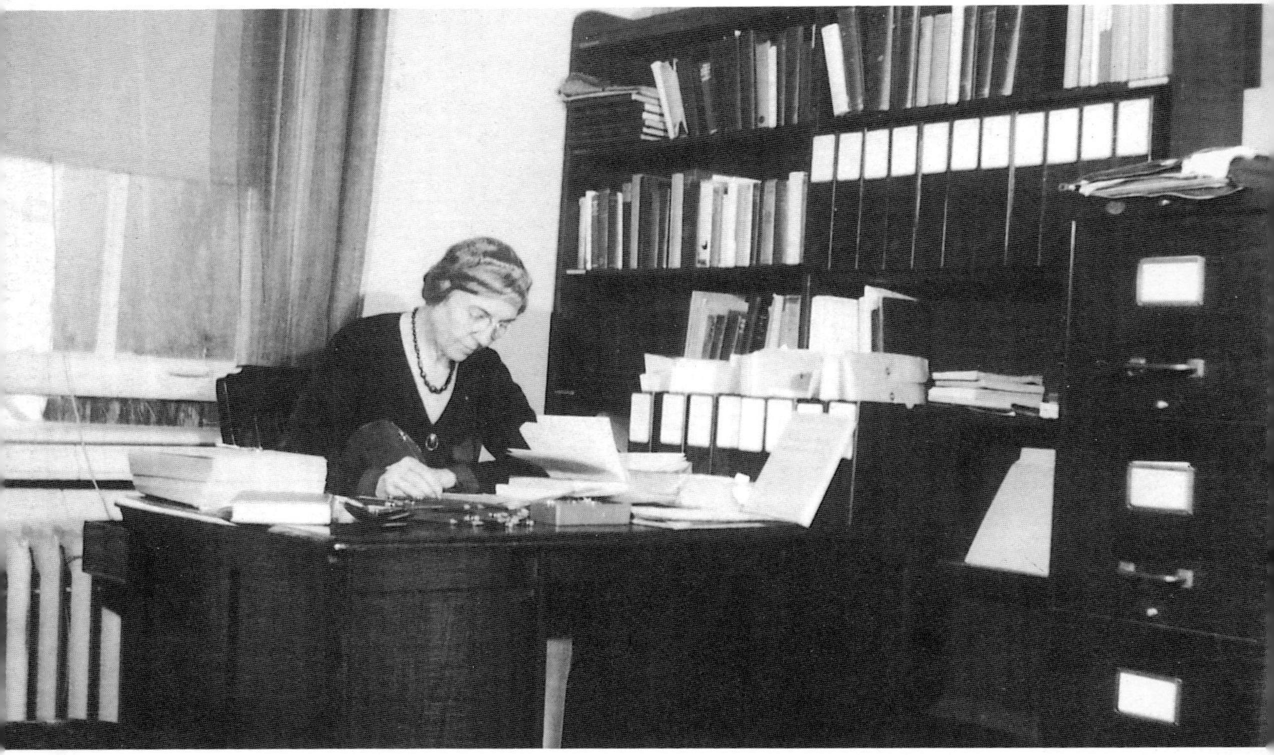

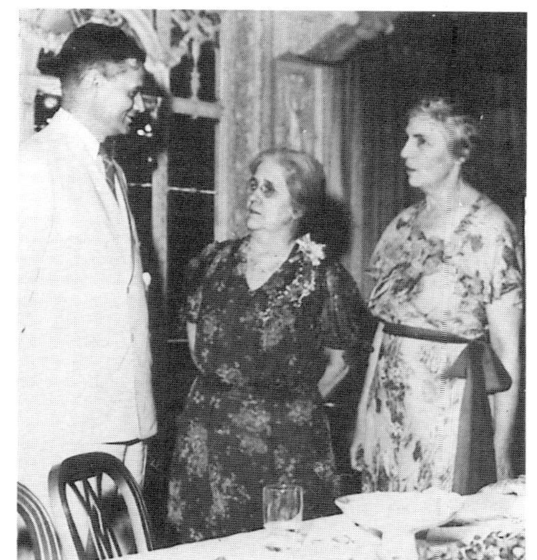

The first Borden Awards for distinction in nutrition research presented at the annual meeting of the American Home Economics Association in Pittsburgh, June 1938. W.A. Wentworth of the Borden Company (left) with 1937 award recipient Dr. Amy L. Daniels of the University of Iowa (center) and 1938 award recipient Dr. Lydia J. Roberts (right). Photo courtesy of Special Collections, Vanderbilt Medical Center Library, Nashville.

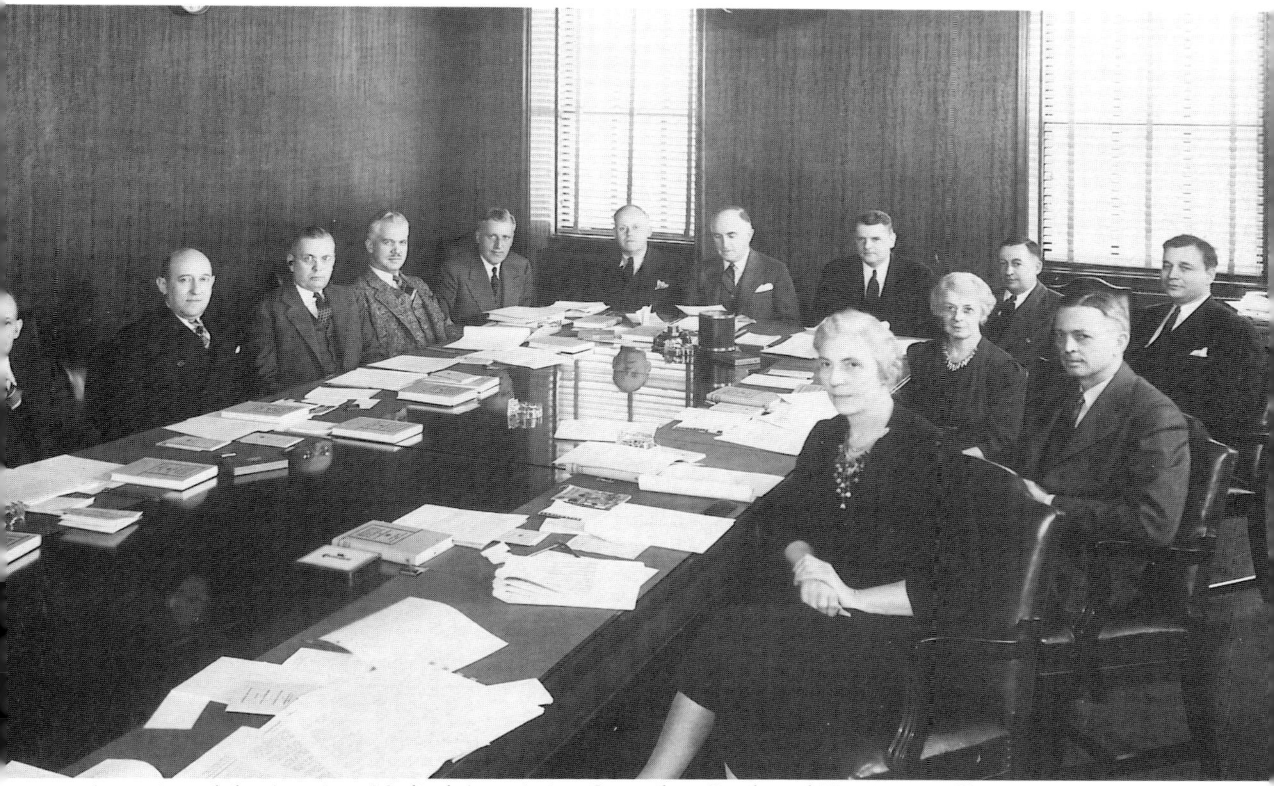

A meeting of the American Medical Association Council on Foods and Nutrition in Chicago, 1940. Lydia Roberts is in the foreground; other participants are (left to right): unidentified, Morris Fishbein, George Cowgill, unidentified, Russell M. Wilder, Howard B. Lewis, J. S. McLester, Franklin Bing, P. N. Leech, Tom D. Spies, Mary S. Rose, and P. C. Jeans. Photo courtesy Special Collections, Vanderbilt Medical Center Library, Nashville.

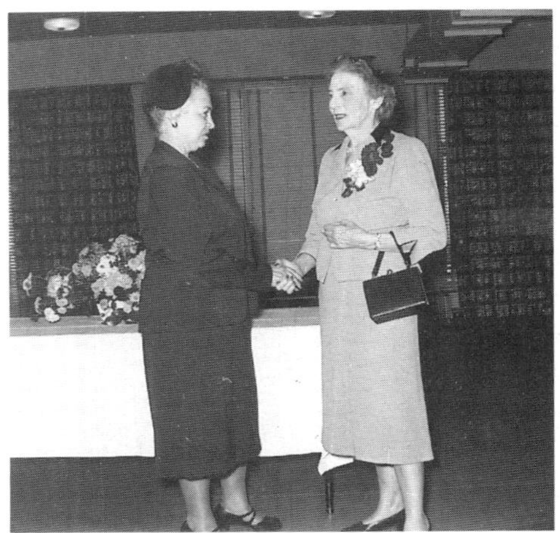

Lydia Roberts (right) with Dr. Miriam E. Lowenberg, marking Dr. Roberts's receiving an honorary membership in Omicron Nu in 1952. Photo courtesy Dr. Miriam E. Lowenberg.

Doña Elena, Puerto Rico, in 1957, at the start of the project to raise the standard of living of families in the area. Photo courtesy Comité de Conferencias Lydia J. Roberts, Río Piedras, Puerto Rico.

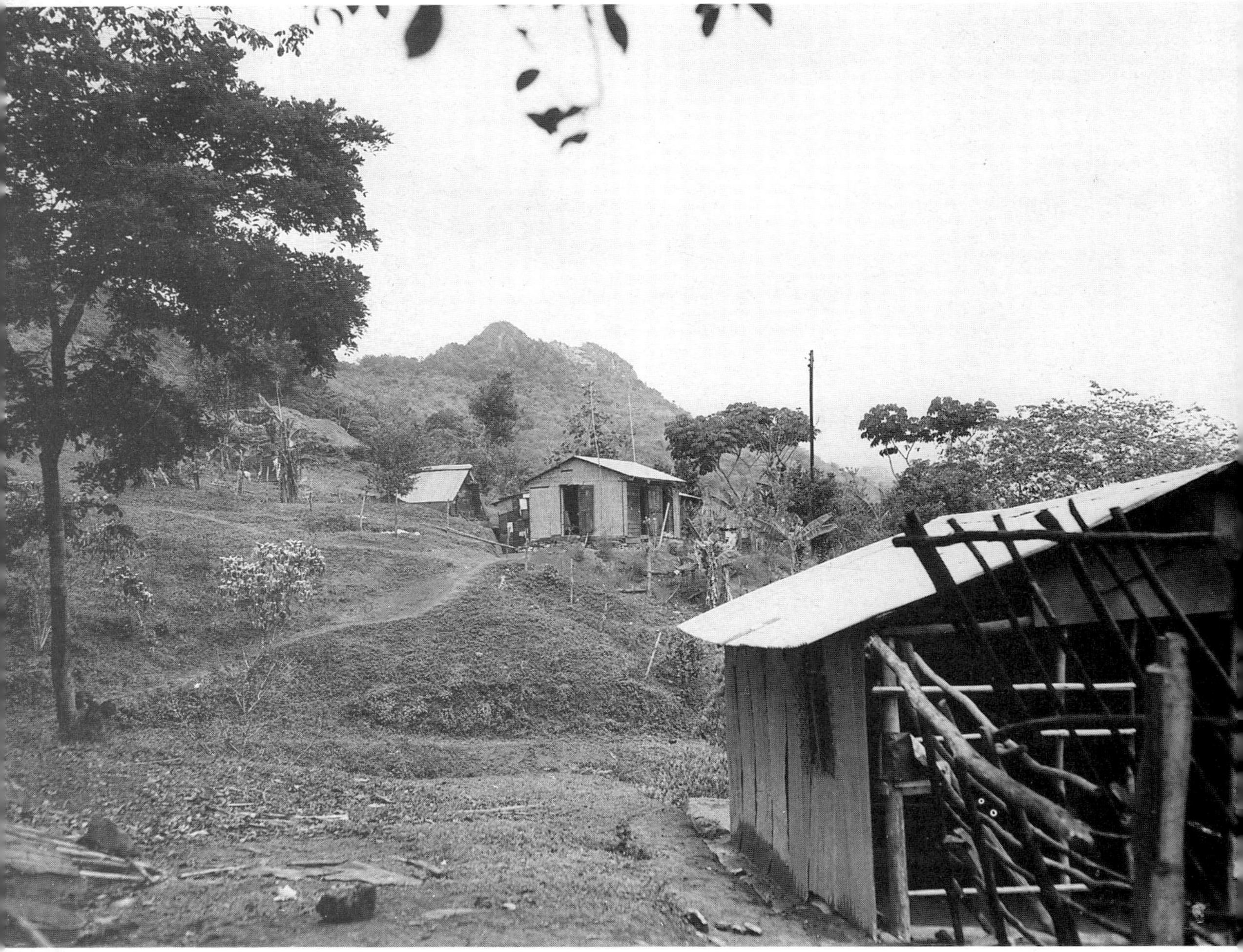

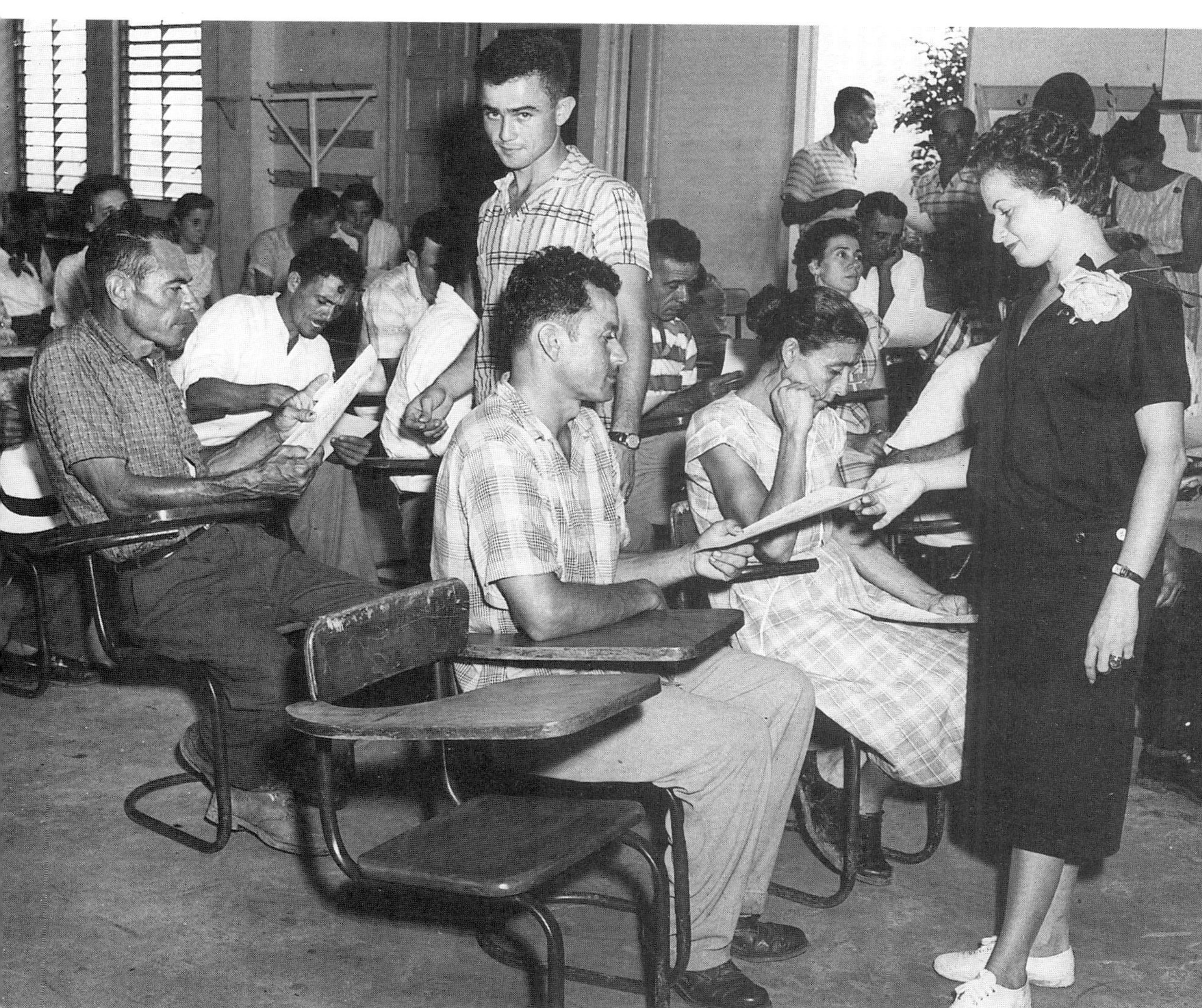

Alejandro (standing center) and Carmen Luz Santiago (standing right) at a meeting at the school, Dona Elena. Photo courtesy Comité de Conferencias Lydia J. Roberts, Río Piedras, Puerto Rico.

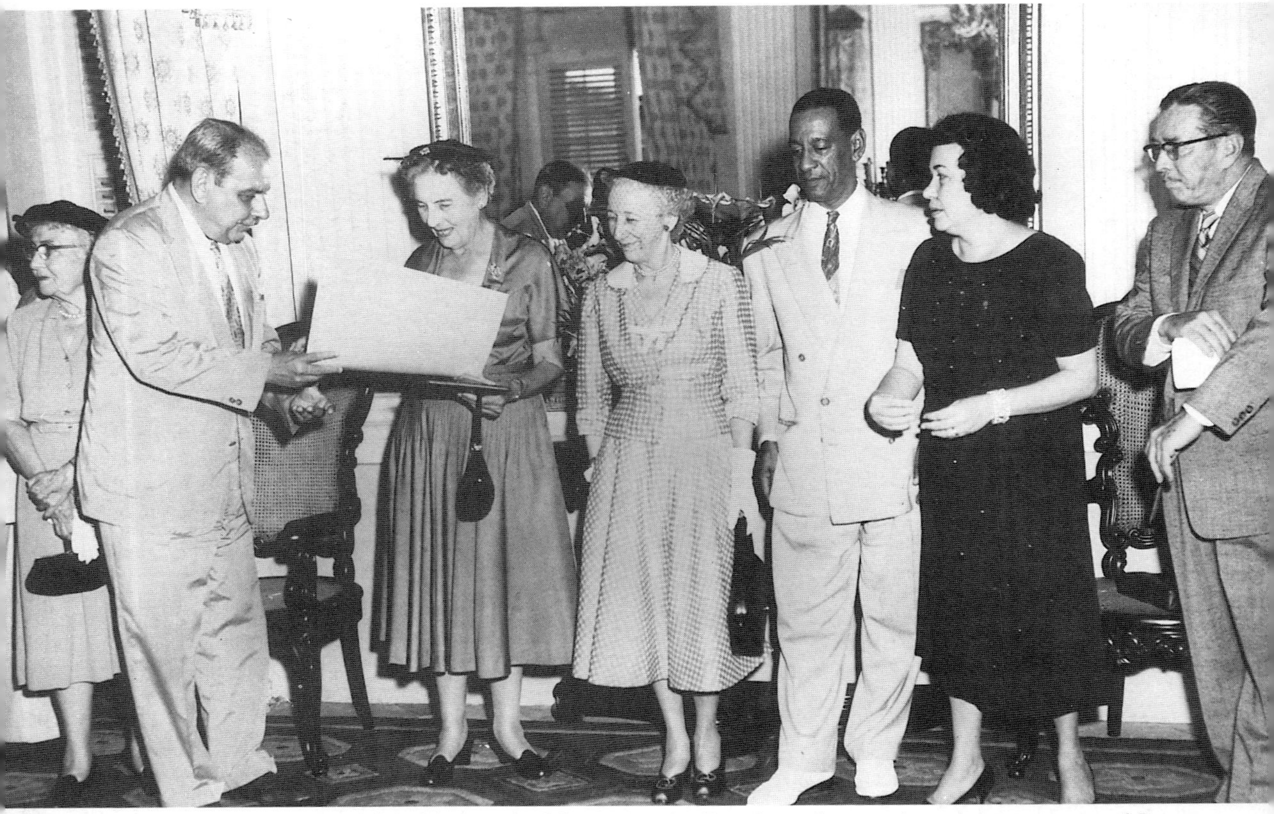

The Marshall Field Award celebration at La Fortaleza, the mansion of the governor of Puerto Rico, 1957. Governor Luis Muñoz Marín presented Dr. Roberts with a certificate naming her Exemplary Citizen of the Commonwealth of Puerto Rico. Also participating in the occasion were Lillian Roberts (far left); Ethel Austin Martin; Ernesto Ramos, president of the Puerto Rico House of Representatives; Inez Muñoz Marín; and Dr. Juan Pono, secretary of health of Puerto Rico. Photo courtesy Special Collections, Vanderbilt Medical Center Library, Nashville.

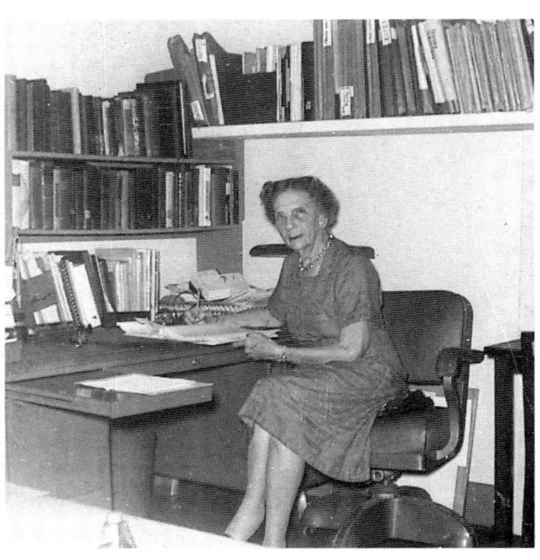

Lydia Roberts in her office at the University of Puerto Rico, Río Piedras, December 1961. Photo by Luis Berrios, courtesy Comité de Conferencias Lydia J. Roberts, Río Piedras, Puerto Rico.

Carmen Luz Santiago measuring child at school in Doña Elena. Photo courtesy Thelma Dreis.

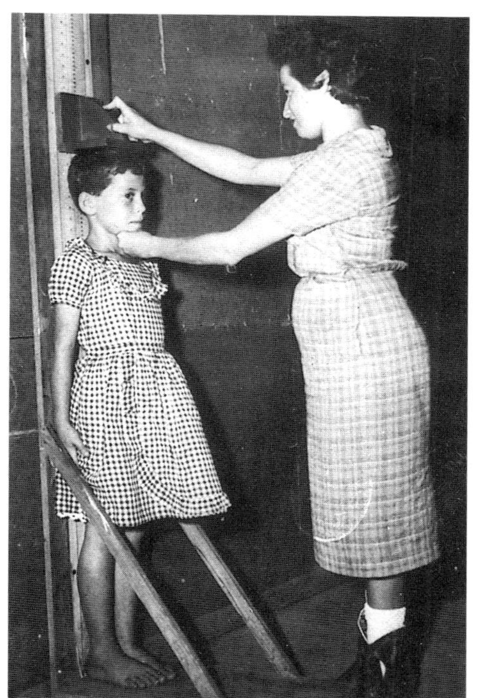

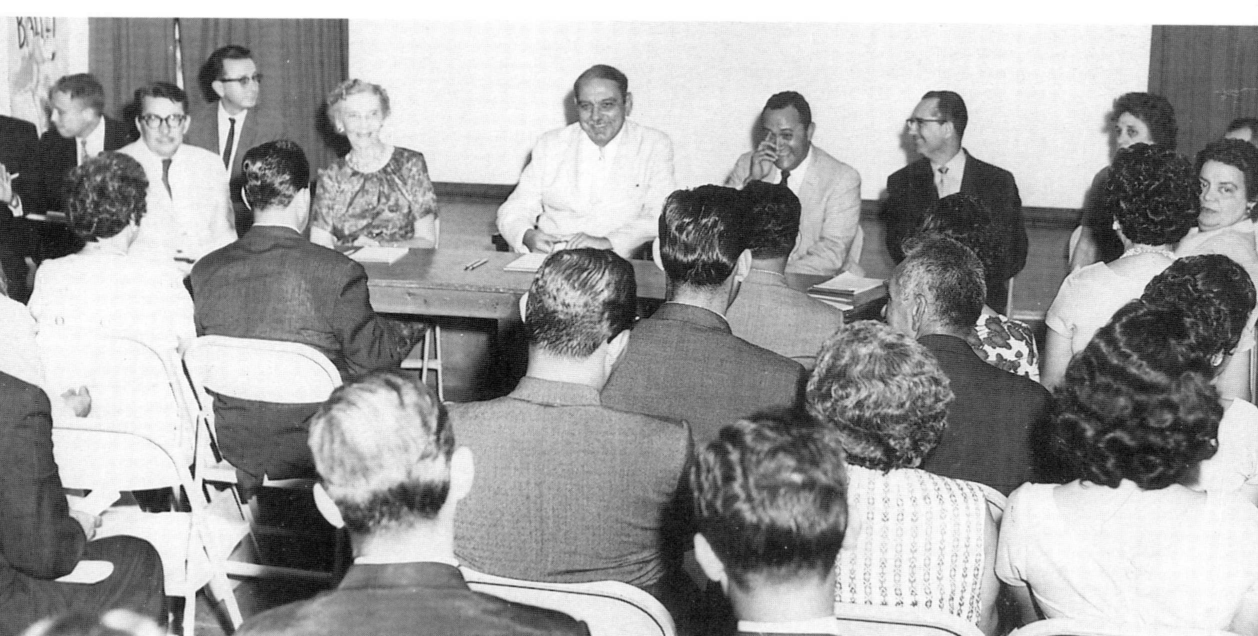

Lydia Roberts with Governor Luis Muñoz Marín in July 1960, when the governor appointed Dr. Roberts chairman of the new Commission for Improvement of Isolated Communities. Photo courtesy Departamento de Estado, Estado Libre Associado de Puerto Rico and the Comité de Conferencias Lydia J. Roberts, Río Piedras, Puerto Rico.

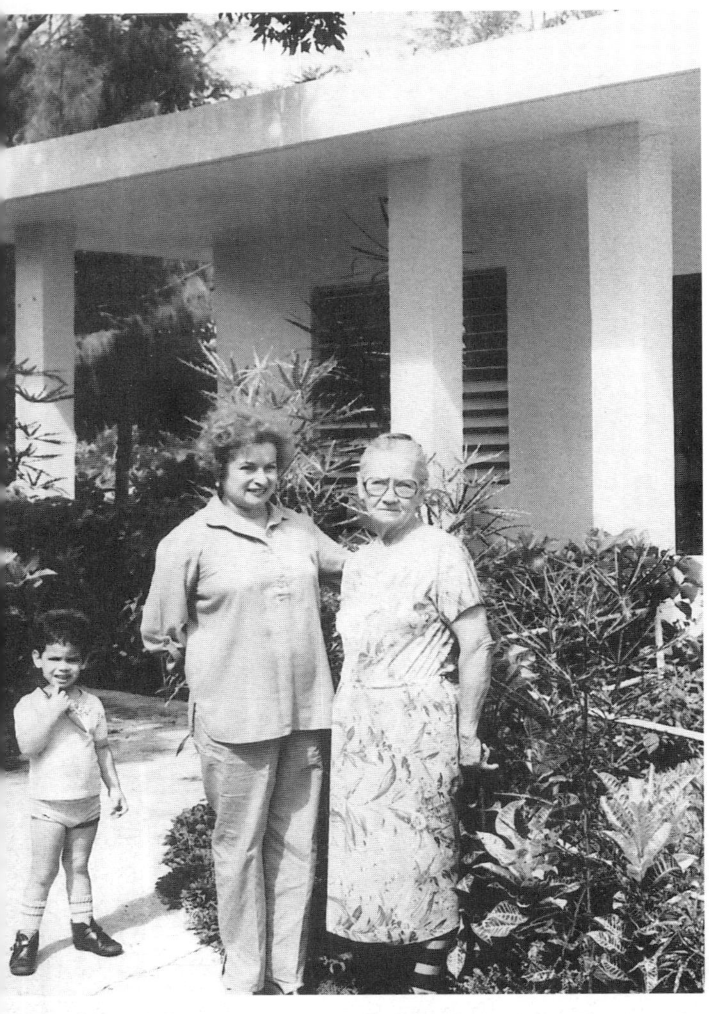

Carmen Luz Santiago de Ramos and Doña Conchita Díaz in front of the Díaz home, Doña Elena, 1986.

Doña Elena in 1960 and 1961, showing one result of the area improvement project: a new house adjoining the old. Photo courtesy Comité de Conferencias Lydia J. Roberts, Río Piedras, Puerto Rico.

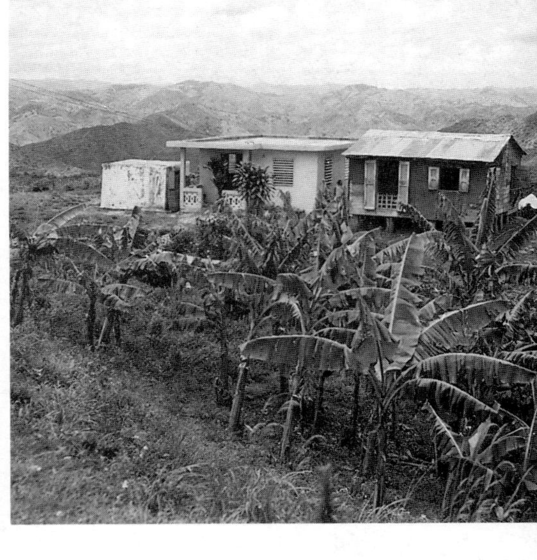

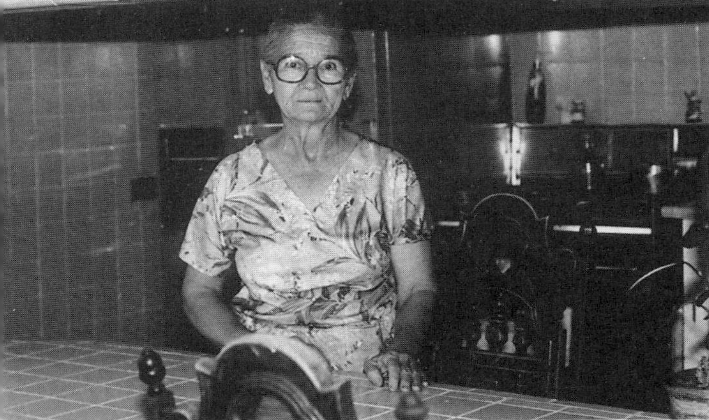

Doña Conchita Díaz in her kitchen, Doña Elena, 1986.

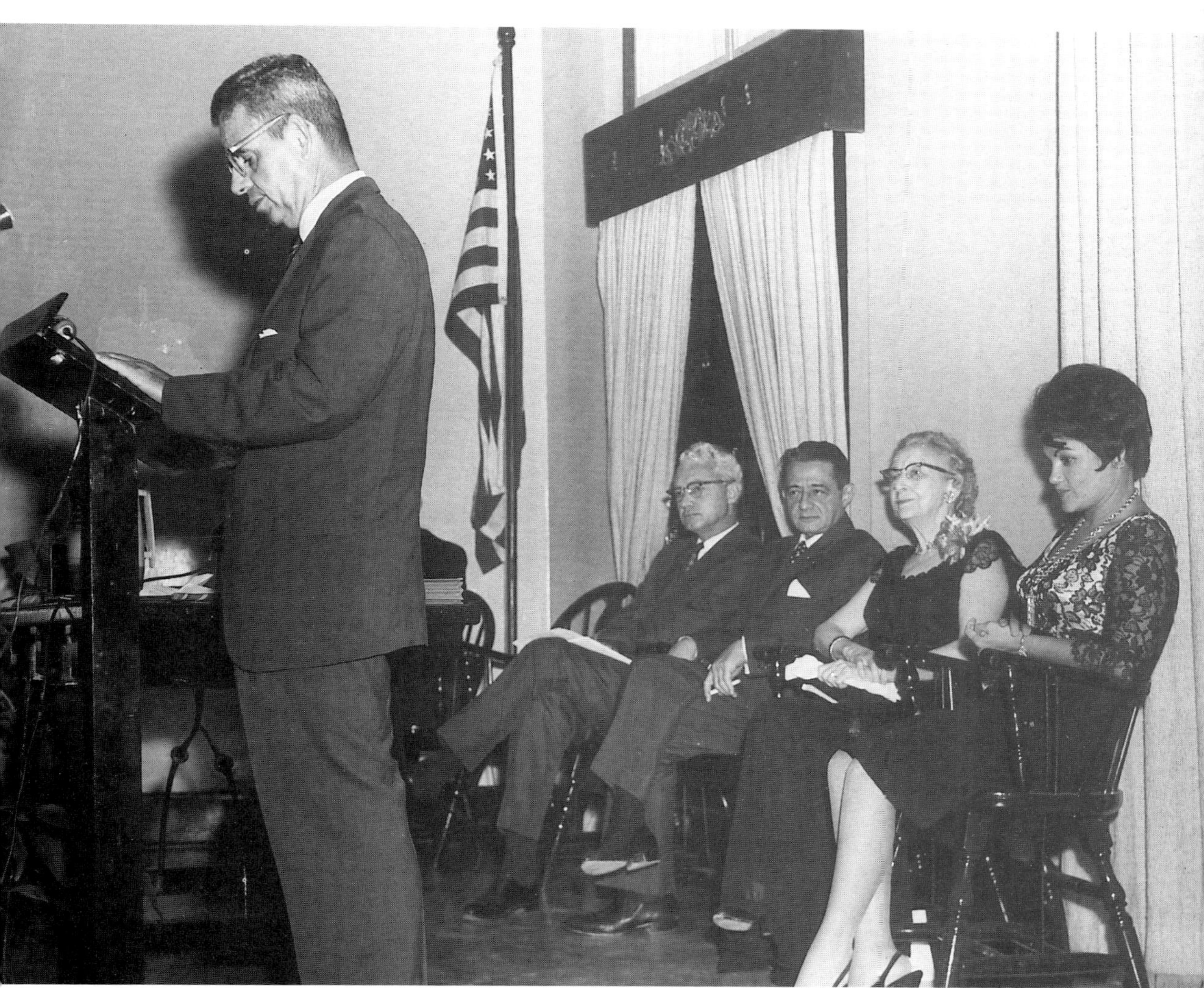

First Lydia J. Roberts Memorial Lecture at the University of Puerto Rico, San Juan, 1966. Dr. Conrado Asenjo at podium introducing speaker Dr. William J. Darby (seated left). Alsc seated (left to right), Jaime Benítez, chancellor of the University; Ethel Austin Martin; and Ruth Davila Fogleman, chair of the lecture committee. Photo courtesy Comité de Conferencias Lydia J. Roberts, Río Piedras, Puerto Rico.

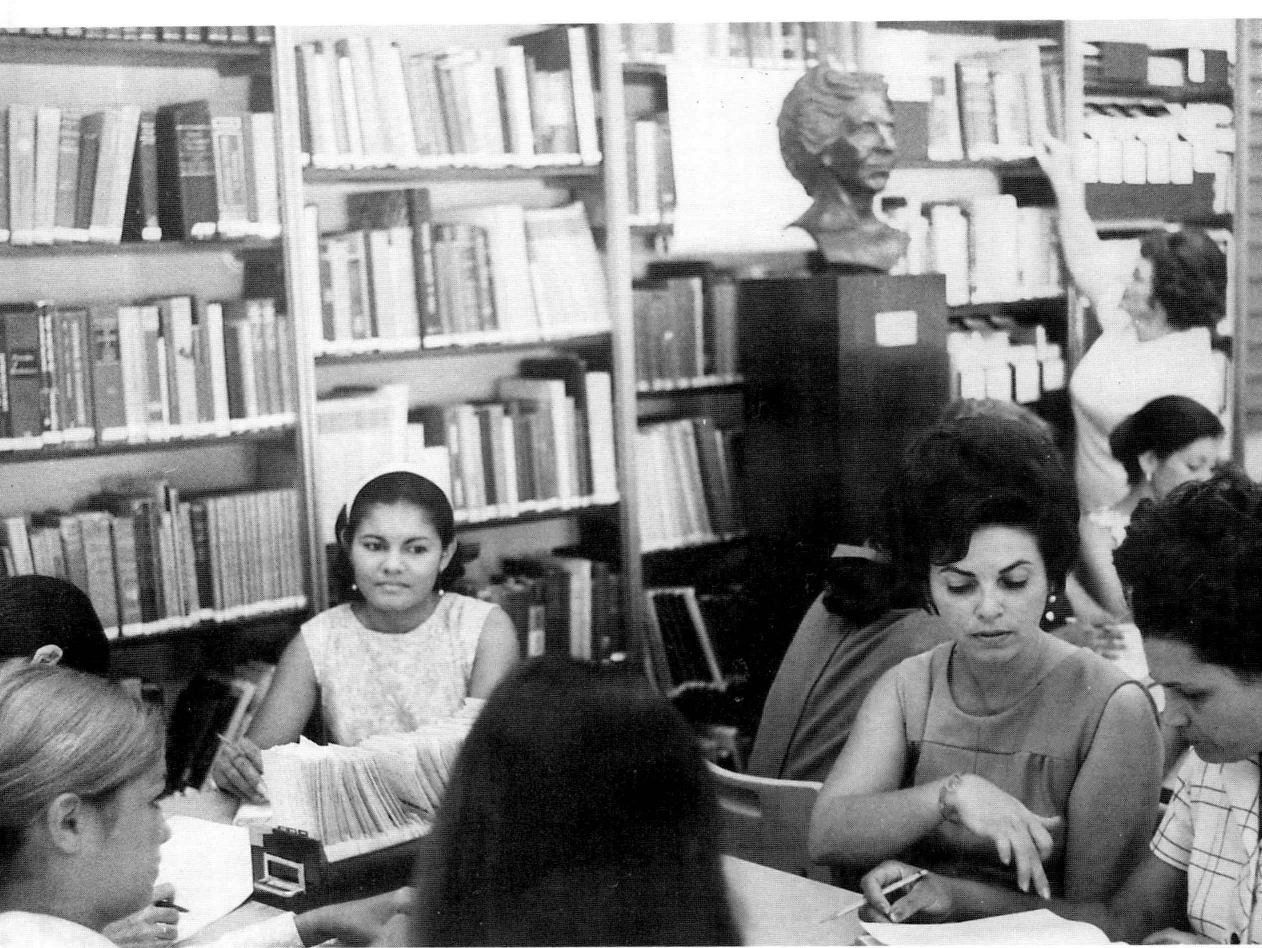

Sala Roberts, University of Puerto Rico School of Home Economics, Río Piedras. Study room also houses audiovisual equipemnt and materials. Photo courtesy Comité de Conferencias Lydia J. Roberts, Río Piedras, Puerto Rico.

CHAPTER 7

An Island Is Reached

Lydia Roberts's third career began during wartime, as had her second. In 1918, when she joined the staff of the University of Chicago, a major concern had been the physical condition of young men in the armed forces. In the early 1940s, with war clouds gathering again, many of the young men being drafted or volunteering for military duty showed the same picture. In 1918 nutrition was a new field. The relationship between food intake and certain physical problems was only beginning to be identified. In the 1940s the picture was clearer, and the methods of dealing with it were better defined. There was much more awareness of the importance of good nutrition and of providing adequate food supplies for everyone, not just the armed forces. If war clouds ever have a silver lining, the one for World War II certainly would include the progress made in developing a yardstick for nutrition needs and in initiating nutrition programs for civilians as well as for the armed forces. Included among the wartime programs were the development of K rations for field use by the military, initiation of nutrient enrichment and fortification of certain basic foods, and rationing of foods in short supply to secure more equitable distribution. Some of these programs, such as the enrichment of cereals and the fortification of margarine, became permanent.

As a result of the concern over nutrition, the Nutrition Service was established in the Federal Security Agency and M. L. Wilson, director of the Federal Extension Service, was appointed as director. The Nutrition Service was devoted chiefly to civilian needs. Nutrition committees were organized at federal, state, and local levels of government. The committees' basic purpose was to promote nutrition education and thereby improve the nutritional status of people. The committee members were representatives of public agencies with activities related to nutrition.

It was at Director Wilson's request that Dr. Roberts had spent two months in 1942 studying the nutritional problems of the southern United States and the work of the various state committees and their constituent agencies in meeting those problems. Now he wanted the same kind of information for Puerto Rico.*

In compliance with Director Wilson's request that Dr. Roberts familiarize herself with the nutrition situation in Puerto Rico, she spent six weeks traveling throughout the island with her hostess and former student, Esther Seijo, extension nutrition specialist. They covered almost all the main roads, saw the country and the people. Dr. Roberts carried a map with her on which she recorded their travels. It was dog-eared and well marked at the end of six weeks! During the course of these travels Dr. Roberts talked with various agency leaders,

> *observing the problems they faced and their methods of dealing with them. . . . I went with extension workers to visit rural homes of all economic levels, attended meetings of adults and 4-H clubs, and talked with specialists in the different areas. I had similar experiences with workers in the Farm Security Administration, the School Lunch Program, the Milk Stations, the schools, especially departments of Home Economics and Vocational Agriculture, the W.P.A., the P.R.A.A., the Health Department.*[1]

Altogether it seems obvious that Dr. Roberts's first visit to Puerto Rico afforded her a fairly informed assessment of the nutrition problems of the island.

On her return from Puerto Rico, Dr. Roberts reported her observations to Director Wilson. She had found widespread undernutrition. He asked her what could be done about it. "My only constructive suggestion was that some improvement could be effected by a workshop for leaders in the various agencies, to help them see how better nutrition could be attained by wiser use of available resources. This appealed to Mr. Wilson as something he could do, and he agreed to finance a nutrition workshop in Puerto Rico, if I would come to direct it. . . ."[1]

In June 1943, Dr. Roberts returned to Puerto Rico to conduct her first nutrition workshop on the island. The workshop was the logical method for her to use in Puerto Rico. The procedures had been tested and developed in the workshops in Chicago and had been in use since the first workshop in 1940. Using these same methods, the Puerto Rican participants could evaluate the nutritional shortcomings of the island's people and seek means of dealing with them.

The first workshop was sponsored by the Puerto Rico Nutrition Committee and was held at the University of Puerto Rico, 1 through 30 June. Funds for the workshop were provided by the Nutrition and Food Conservation Branch of the Food Distribution Administration, the federal agency that assisted state nutrition committees. The purpose of the workshop was to bring together leaders from

*Puerto Rico was initially a U.S. territory, with the governor appointed by the president. Puerto Rico elected its first governor in 1948. The island became the Commonwealth of Puerto Rico in 1952.

agencies concerned with nutrition in Puerto Rico and to help them work together on the problem of developing and coordinating more effective activities for improving the state of nutrition of the people of the island.[1]

Sixty-seven people participated in the workshop including extension agents (agriculture and home economics), supervisors and teachers of home economics and agriculture, school-lunch supervisors, and elementary and secondary teachers. Three people from the Virgin Islands attended: a school superintendent, a secondary-school teacher, and the state supervisor of the Home Management Section of the Farm Security Administration.[2] It was a well-selected group of people. In later years some of them held high-level jobs in government and administration and were able to assist Dr. Roberts in her future activities.

The schedule for each day of the workshop opened with a session on nutrition information. Then followed a discussion period on nutrition needs and on methods and resources for dealing with them. This session included group and roundtable discussions and sometimes lectures. In the afternoons participants worked individually or in small groups on problems of special interest to them. To facilitate the operation of the workshop, committees were formed: summarizing, program, social activity, field trips, and publicity. No opportunity for nutrition education was lost. Milk breaks replaced coffee breaks. Lunches featured native foods of good nutrition quality, such as the *calabaza*, a squash of high vitamin A content.[2]

A notable outcome of the workshop was the reorganization of the Puerto Rico Nutrition Committee, which had been formed a year or two earlier. It had been active for a while, but was inactive at the time of the workshop. Now plans were made for the committee to carry out ideas developed in the workshop. As the story of Dr. Roberts's participation in Puerto Rico unfolds, the lead role of the rejuvenated Nutrition Committee in a number of significant programs will become evident.

A person who became aware of Dr. Roberts at this time and who was to be a staunch supporter and loyal friend was Jaime Benítez, chancellor of the University of Puerto Rico. He invited her to return to the university to assist with the reorganization of the curriculum of the Department of Home Economics. In considering the invitation, Dr. Roberts wrote to Marie Vestal, the head of the department, asking if her assistance would be welcome. Marie Vestal replied with a cordial yes, whereupon Dr. Roberts accepted the invitation and returned to the university early in 1944 for a two-month stay.

In developing the new curriculum, the faculty agreed that they should start from scratch "and plan a program suited to the needs of Puerto Rico, irrespective of what had been done previously. Since the purpose of home economics is the improvement of living in homes, it was decided that we should first know what those needs are."[1] The faculty set about gathering this information, using the published material available and their own observations. Although few accurate data were available on Puerto Rican living conditions, the faculty worked out a program of courses that, they believed, would prepare students to deal with the types of problems they might encounter. This program included at least one basic course in each major aspect of family life. Home economics courses were needed in some previously unrecognized areas: the socioeconomic problems of Puerto Rican families, family health, bacteriology, family relations, and home food production. Dr. Roberts also made recommendations concerning staff and salaries. One innovative idea included a proposal for a 20-acre farm home where students could experience rural life. The latter proposal was approved verbally by the chancellor, but was never implemented. The new curriculum was adopted, however, and the recommendations concerning the faculty were carried out.

After the two months spent working on the curriculum and developing the creative new approach to home economics in Puerto Rico, Dr. Roberts returned to the University of Chicago. By then, only a few months remained before her retirement in June. Undoubtedly, the months were busy, with many loose ends to be tied up and many preparations to be made for turning the department affairs over to the new head, Dr. Thelma Porter. Perhaps there were many times, however, that Dr. Roberts, when putting away the old, must have thought about the new programs in Puerto Rico that she had helped to develop. With her feeling for the future, that work was probably of as much or more interest to her than the job of laying down the reins for someone else to take over.

It must have been a pleasant and welcome event when Chancellor Benítez invited her to return to the University of Puerto Rico. She agreed to go for six months, to arrive in November 1944 and stay until June 1945. She continued to work on the new curriculum, developed syllabi for courses, and thoroughly enjoyed Puerto Rico and its climate. Soon after her arrival (it was 25 November 1944, 7:45 AM) she wrote, "I am sitting by an open window with all doors and windows open, the temperature is 75 °F, we have another nice day. And what days! The skies are the bluest blue you ever saw, with great piles of soft billowy clouds. . . . And the ocean: well I can't describe it."

Dr. Roberts's working relationship with Chancellor Benítez was most gratifying. She was embarrassed, she wrote, "by the things the Chancellor thinks I know and can do. Today, he sent me to check on plans for a new dormitory for girls and he says every suggestion I make goes, and then he'll put all the blame (or credit?) on me. I'll have one bit of credit, that I got the kitchen on the same floor as the dining room . . . I may slip down the bean stalk, but now my stock is high."

There was even some time for writing during the six-month stay. Dr. Roberts, a natural-born educator, did not closet herself and write—she formed a "little writing club" among the faculty. They wrote booklets about the life of an imaginary family. This family's living was a synthesis drawn from their own. Each booklet described some improvement the family was making. Dr. Roberts enjoyed the writing. She described it as "so much fun," and, "I don't want to do anything else. But I let myself do it only at odd times as a treat."

Back in Chicago, after spending six months in Puerto Rico, Dr. Roberts was visited by Chancellor Benítez one day. He asked her to join the faculty of the Department of Home Economics and to serve as its head. Marie Vestal planned to resign the position at the end of the semester in December 1945. Dr. Roberts had a deep-seated interest in the curriculum for home economics, which she had helped to develop. She was interested in Chancellor Benítez's invitation. However, there were certain prerequisites for accepting it. She would consider it "only if a strong forward looking program of development were contemplated." To her satisfaction, the stipulations were met. She returned to Puerto Rico in January 1946 and became head of the Department of Home Economics. Her third career was officially under way.

REFERENCES

1. Roberts LJ: Review of Activities in Puerto Rico (from February 1943 to January 1951). Submitted to Chancellor Jaime Benítez, University of Puerto Rico, March 1951.
2. Program for Workshop in Community Nutrition. Río Piedras, PR, University of Puerto Rico, June 1943.

CHAPTER 8

The Island Becomes Hers

When Lydia Roberts returned to Puerto Rico in January 1946, something was different. Now she was on "her island," as she was already calling it, not for one month, six weeks, nor six months, but as a permanent member of the faculty of the University of Puerto Rico.

Shortly after her return, an event most pleasing to her occurred: the university granted funds for a research project that she earnestly wished to do—a study of patterns of living in Puerto Rican families. Before her return to Chicago, she had discussed the research with Chancellor Jaime Benítez and had even submitted a plan for it. Findings from the study were needed for the further development of a curriculum in home economics that was realistic to family life. Such information was also essential for program planning by community agencies.

Dr. Roberts threw herself energetically into making plans for the study. She was determined to find out everything she could about Puerto Rican homes at every socioeconomic level. M. L. Wilson, who had been instrumental in Dr. Roberts's first visit to the island, was interested in the project. He sent a staff member from his office to assist. Thelma Dreis was an expert on preparing interview schedules. Selecting a sample representative of the island's population was a major task; selecting and training interviewers was another. Dr. Roberts and Rosa Luisa Stefani, the associate head of the Department of Home Economics, drove to many parts of the island to select interviewers. Their travels brought nature-loving Lydia Roberts her first sight of some of Puerto Rico's beauty—the blooming flamboyants. "They are those gorgeous, spreading trees covered with deep red blossoms," she wrote. "We drove for miles and miles over mountain roads literally aflame with them. It was really breath taking."

The careful planning required for the project occupied Dr. Roberts and her staff for the better part of six months. Then the research got under way. From June to October 1946, approximately 1,000 families were interviewed and the schedules were edited and coded. The data were tabulated during the remaining months of 1946. An account of the project was prepared for publication in 1947.[1] The classic study, *Patterns of Living in Puerto Rican Families,* did not come off the press, however, until the fall of 1949.[2] It was dedicated to Jaime Benítez.

The goal of learning as much as possible about Puerto Rican families was well carried out. *Patterns of Living* contained detailed information on housing, sanitary facilities, household equipment, health habits, medical care, food preferences, food sources, and food consumption. The book was an essential reference for students in the home economics curriculum and for professionals in community agencies. Another prime user was Governor Luis Muñoz Marín, who told a visitor that "he didn't dare prepare new family welfare programs or changes in welfare policies without consulting it."

Along with a strenuous work program, Dr. Roberts found time to get acquainted with Puerto Rico and Puerto Ricans during this, her first full year on the island. There were numerous social events, including a picnic with Chancellor Benítez and his family and a group of their friends at Luquillo Beach. She enjoyed everything about the picnic and wrote a description of the beach:

> *. . . the most beautiful beach I've ever seen. It is a beautifully curved sandy beach with coconut palms going down almost to the water, and with a mountain range in the distance, for background. That landscape with the blue ocean, blue sky, white clouds, yellow sand, and dark mountains is really magnificent.*

Dr. Roberts's description reflects her love for the shores of Lake Michigan around Chicago and in the Indiana Dunes area.

The year 1946 was marked by another workshop—the first of a long series of workshops in Puerto Rico and the Caribbean area. The 1946 workshop, held in June, was for school-lunch managers. Three years later, three workshops for teachers—in nutrition, home improvement, and home food production—were conducted concurrently. In addition, two workshops—one in nutrition and food preparation and the other in elements of clothing—were given to people who taught native handicrafts. It seemed to Dr. Roberts and her co-workers that these teachers "could do much to improve home living if they were taught some of the fundamental material of Home Economics."[1]

All of the 1949 workshops for teachers were repeated in 1950. That year the workshops spread beyond Puerto Rico. Margaret Hockin, rural welfare officer of the Food and Agriculture Organization (FAO), had visited many Caribbean countries and also Puerto Rico, where she learned of Dr. Roberts's workshops. She was impressed, and she proposed that workers from the Caribbean area be allowed to participate. Such a workshop was arranged. Twelve people took part in it: three from Jamaica, two from Trinidad, and one each from Dominica, Grenada, Barbados, British Honduras, British Guiana, Curacao, and Suriname. The university waived tuition, individual countries paid travel expenses, and the United Nations paid for books and lodging. In all of the workshops, Dr. Roberts's down-to-earth, thrifty, practical nature was evident. The procedures used could be adopted in the homes of the children in the teachers' classes. In the nutrition and food-preparation workshop, the participants used measuring devices and cooking utensils that could be created at home, chiefly from cans. In home improvement, cupboards, tables, chairs, and closets were constructed from boxes and barrels. Broken steps and floorboards were mended. Areas around homes were cleaned, and flowers and shrubs were planted.

And surely the practical approach was successful. Margaret Harrington, an FAO officer who visited Puerto Rico that summer, was "favorably impressed with the practical approaches then being used by the staff of the University of Puerto Rico in its programs for rural families." She pointed out that "it was Dr. Roberts who gave the vision and drive for such programs."

But the best report came from Dr. Roberts. She described an incident that had taken place at a joint session of participants in one of the 1949 workshops:

> *A man and his wife whose home had been improved (by the home improvement group) came and told about it. It was wonderful. The woman simply raved about* mi cocina preciosa *[my wonderful kitchen]. She kept bursting out with more things; her enthusiasm was the most telling part. The husband too added most significant points; one, for example, that he had moved the pig pen away from the house.*

Although workshops took up much of Dr. Roberts's attention during this period, she never overlooked "spreading the nutrition gospel" in as many ways as possible. Her skill as a teacher continued to inspire others. She helped to prepare brochures and booklets that told the nutrition story simply and effectively. She made many speeches and took part in many meetings. She involved students as well as staff. Her enjoyment of these activities was shown in a letter written in 1947:

> *Saturday we had an all day session . . . a district Home Economics Association. Mrs. Torres and I and our nutrition students put on three demonstrations of graphic methods of teaching nutrition. We did one on "better rice," one on "better beans" and one on use of native fruits. They were quite effective. I wrote a skit for the first one, and we have been requested to repeat it at the Island meeting in July. So you see I'm up to my old tricks of devising teaching methods.*

Visual aids were not forgotten, either. Among the teaching aids Dr. Roberts helped prepare was a filmstrip on "Puerto Rico's Golden Treasure"—the *calabaza*. It was intended for presentation to rural housewives, and told about the *calabaza*'s nutritive value, different ways of preparing it to increase its use, how to select good ones in the market, and how to grow them in patios or fields. Two hundred copies of this filmstrip were prepared, and they were used throughout the island.[3]

Dr. Roberts encouraged the Puerto Rico Nutrition Committee to develop a simple and effective food chart for teaching good nutrition. The chart was divided into five sections. One section listed "Foods Which Almost Everyone Eats Now." The other four sections showed groups of "Other Food That Everyone Should Eat." The food groups listed were milk; meat, fish, fowl and eggs; "yellows and greens" (native vegetables rich in vitamin A); and fresh native fruits. The chart was colorful and attractive and it adapted easily for use with a flannel board. It also was used all over the island, and in time became a guide for preparing food charts for other Latin American countries.[3]

The six years between 1946 and 1952, when Dr. Roberts was head of the Department of Home Economics at the University of Puerto Rico, were fruitful. Dr. Roberts produced the classic study of how Puerto Ricans live, and people in a position to do something about the conditions paid attention to the findings. Dr. Roberts made other significant contributions to the betterment of living of the people on the island, and her methods were attracting attention; they were models.

REFERENCES

1. Roberts LJ: Review of Activities in Puerto Rico (from February 1943 to January 1951). Submitted to Chancellor Jaime Benítez, University of Puerto Rico, March 1951.
2. Roberts LJ, Stefani RL: *Patterns of Living in Puerto Rican Families.* Río Piedras, PR, University of Puerto Rico, 1949.
3. Roberts LJ: A basic food pattern for Puerto Rico. *J Am Diet Assoc* 30:1097, 1954.

CHAPTER 9

Helping Her Island's People

Lydia Roberts held that home economics should have a part in community activities aimed at improving home and family living. She adhered to this tenet even more than ever in Puerto Rico.

The Puerto Rican government consulted with Dr. Roberts a number of times. The government was seeking to achieve a better life for its people, and Dr. Roberts was asked to participate in this effort. Another of her continuing community services was with the Puerto Rico Nutrition Committee. As a member of the committee, she energetically took part in its programs.

The first of the government's requests came in 1946, early in Dr. Roberts's leadership of the Department of Home Economics. The Minimum Wage Board asked for a minimum budget for white-collar workers, to set minimum wages for this class of worker. Members of the Department of Home Economics collaborated to put the budget together. At about the same time, the Social Welfare Division of the Department of Health asked for assistance in drawing up a minimum food budget for relief families. Department members provided these budgets.

Availability of dry skim milk for human consumption and consumer acceptance of it were problems in which Dr. Roberts became decisively involved. By Puerto Rican law, dry skim milk, an imported product, could be brought into the country only for animal food, not for human consumption. To assure that the product would not be used as an adulterant, green coloring was added to it. Of course, the law had to be amended if dry skim milk were to be accepted by consumers. This was accomplished, and the color requirement was deleted. Following the passage of the amendment, the government engaged in a tremendous campaign to tell people about dry skim milk—that it was a food for humans, and that it was of superior nutritive value. All agencies with a nutrition connection took part in the campaign, which extended to all parts of the island.

Dry skim milk needed to be available in the marketplace in package sizes convenient for the consumer. The Nutrition Committee tackled the package-size problem in 1948. The thrust of the committee's effort was to encourage producers to market dry skim milk not only in acceptably sized packages, but also at a price about half that of an equivalent amount of whole milk in any form. The milk companies were reluctant to take the risk.

The dry-skim-milk project interested recently elected Governor Luis Muñoz Marín and his wife, Inez Mendoza de Muñoz Marín. Dr. Roberts tells of their concern:

> *I was in their home for dinner one night with a few others. . . . My being invited to dinner was all on account of dry skim milk. Mrs. Muñoz asked some of us to come in the afternoon to talk about it. Then the next day, she asked me to come to dinner to explain it to Muñoz. She had the commissioners of Agriculture, Education, and Health also. I taught them about dry skim milk. The next day we were all invited to come at 4:00 o'clock and work on the problem, and again have dinner. I feel quite "chummy" now with the governor, his wife, and cabinet. It's all because I'm interested in what they are. . . bettering the lot of the common people.*[1]

During the time when the dry-skim-milk producers were pondering the nutrition-committee proposal, Robert Rosenbaum, an official of the Borden Milk Company, visited Puerto Rico. While there he conferred with Dr. Roberts and learned of the Nutrition Committee's desire to have dry skim milk available in Puerto Rico at a reasonable price. He suggested that Dr. Roberts go to Chicago and plead the case for dry skim milk with the Borden Company's board of directors. She followed his suggestion, and the Borden Company decided to market dry skim milk in Puerto Rico at the price requested by the Nutrition Committee. The dry-skim-milk project was clearly a great success.

Then in 1950, Governor Muñoz Marín made an urgent request for a plan of priorities for imported foodstuffs in case restrictions should become necessary. Dr. Roberts felt this to be "a most responsible task." Josefina Royo and Rosa Marina Torres of the home economics faculty collaborated with her on this job. As a basis for their calculations, they used the import figures of the previous year, an estimate of home production of food, an approximation of the nutrient needs of the population, and a computation of the nutrient value of the foodstuffs expected to be available. The foods to be imported were divided into six groups—ranging from those that could be cut off with no nutritive loss to the basic food supply to those that should be retained at almost any cost. The latter group included rice, beans, lard, codfish, flour, cereals, and milk. The nutrients per capita contributed by this group of imported foods was computed, and recommendations were made for a home-food-production program to supplement it.

The report was accepted and priorities were established. As was to be expected, the report aroused the ire of certain special groups. However, Lydia Roberts had nothing personal to gain from her recommendations. The only special interest she had was the Puerto Rican people themselves. The next year, in 1951, Governor Muñoz Marín appointed a committee to survey the nutrition situation in the Insular Penitentiary. Members of the committee, in addition to Dr. Roberts, were Dr. Esther Seijo de Zayas, extension nutrition specialist, and Antonio Fernández of the School Lunch Program. The committee was appointed following an uprising in the prison, claimed to have been staged because of the poor food and inadequate equipment in the kitchen and dining room. The committee members were given the responsibility of determining if the claims made by the inmates were defensible and of making recommendations for improvement if needed.

The committee carried out extensive observations and submitted a report to the governor on 26 February 1951. The report stated that the food itself was probably not the cause of the revolt, for it was similar to what most of the men had been accustomed to in their own homes. However, the committee felt that the methods of preparation and the details of service could be legitimate causes for complaint. For example, there were only 300 spoons available for 2,400 inmates at the time of the committee's inspection. The spoons were washed—in cold water—several times during the course of meal service, but some of the men had to eat with their fingers. Specific recommendations were made concerning ways to improve food production and service, as well as the nutritive value of the food, at only a small increase in cost. The committee pointed out, however, that considerable improvement could be made without any increase in the cash allowance.[2]

In addition to making the report to the governor, the committee members met with the attorney general, the warden, and other officials of the Department of Justice to discuss the report. Dr. Roberts described the meeting:

> *They adopted all our recommendations, appropriated $20,000 to improve the kitchen and the feeding situation in general, approved our recommendation for a dietitian for all penal institutions, etc. They did this because the Governor read the report, marked all of the important suggestions and told them to do something very soon.*

As a result of this study, the committee was asked to survey the other penal institutions. Later the investigation extended to all Health Department institutions. In all, about 20 units were surveyed. Dr. Roberts's reaction to this strenuous and extensive responsibility: "a most interesting and enlightening experience."

Although nutrition programs were of major concern, they were not the only programs in which Dr. Roberts was involved. One public service was the establishment of Community Sewing Centers. Only a small number of families owned sewing machines at that time.[3] Sewing centers, where women could go to work and receive any assistance they needed, represented one solution. Because the members of the Department of Home Economics believed such a program could be helpful to families of low and moderate incomes, they were glad to cooperate.

Inez Muñoz Marín took a special interest in the project and served as honorary chairman of the committee established to develop it. The project was started in 1950. In Dr. Roberts's 1951 report to Chancellor Benítez, she said, "Mrs. Muñoz proposed that the Committee go all out for such a center in every one of the some 800 barrios. . . .great strides have already been made toward this goal."[4]

One of Dr. Roberts's major achievements for Puerto Rico had to do with a program for the enrichment of rice. Puerto Rico had a law requiring the enrichment of flour; however, the main cereal consumed in Puerto Rico is rice, not flour. At Dr. Roberts's suggestion, Dr. Robert R. Williams was invited by the Nutrition Committee to visit Puerto Rico. Dr. Williams, who isolated and later synthesized thiamin, was an enthusiastic advocate of rice enrichment. Dr. Roberts had spoken to Governor and Mrs. Muñoz Marín about Dr. Williams's visit, and they invited him to be their guest at La Fortaleza, the governor's palace. In planning Dr. Williams's visit, Dr. Roberts arranged for him to give a public lecture on enrichment and she saw to it that he had the opportunity to confer with physicians, rice importers, and members of the Nutrition Committee.[4] Apparently his schedule was full—but in a letter describing his visit, Dr. Roberts was careful to point out that she did save some of his time for seeing the island!

Dr. Williams's visit started the enrichment ball rolling in Puerto Rico. After he left, Governor Muñoz Marín set up a committee to follow the matter and to make recommendations about enrichment legislation. Dr. Roberts was made chairman of the Rice Enrichment Committee. The first action of the committee was to ask the Commissioner of Health to require institutions under his charge to use enriched rice. The order was issued, and the use of enriched rice was started. School-lunch programs under the Department of Public Instruction, and the penal institutions under the Department of Justice, also began to use enriched rice. The use of enriched rice by all government institutions assured a sizable demand for the product.

Things seemed to be moving along smoothly when problems arose with the millers. They asked higher prices for the enriched rice than for the unenriched rice, and they claimed that they were unable to ensure delivery. Dr. Roberts and her committee countered this increased-price claim with a few calculations showing that the enrichment would add less than one-fourth cent per pound to the retail price of rice, if the cost of the necessary equipment was amortized over several years.[5]

A rice-enrichment bill was introduced into the Puerto Rico House of Representatives. The following circumstances may have contributed to its defeat. The California Rice Growers Association supplied much of Puerto Rico's rice. A large order of enriched rice supplied by the association for use in public institutions and for distribution to needy families had been enriched by the parboiling method. When cooked, this product bore little resemblance to rice familiar to Puerto Ricans; it had a distinct yellowish color. A climate of dissatisfaction with enriched rice was created even though the enrichment requested in the bill was by premix and not by parboiling.

The governor recalled the rice-enrichment bill. A new bill was introduced later. In the meantime, the Rice Enrichment Committee worked at informing the legislators of the difference in nutritive value between enriched and unenriched rice. The University of Puerto Rico School of Medicine conducted feeding tests with experimental animals to show the difference between the two rices. The superior growth of the rats fed enriched rice was emphasized by Dr. Roberts, who said, "These could be children, you know."[5] The committee cited studies that disclosed that the diets of Puerto Ricans were often deficient in thiamin, niacin, and iron, the nutrients added in enrichment. Medical reports were compiled that showed evidence of deficiencies of these three nutrients in the Puerto Rican population.

When the next rice-enrichment bill was introduced, each legislator had a packet of scientific information on his desk providing evidence for support of the bill. The Rice Enrichment Committee had placed it there.

The account of the fate of this rice-enrichment bill must be told in Dr. Roberts's words:

> *My most exciting experience this week was helping to give a push through the House for our enriched rice bill. We thought all was going well with it when we learned that the Chamber of Commerce had written house members that they should not pass it, because of excessive cost; because equipment could not be obtained to make it, etc., etc.,. . . By the time we had learned about it, the House had voted it down. . . .But through the governor's secretary, we got them to agree to reconsider it. Then six of us went to the legislature and spent the afternoon, 2:00 to 7:00* PM, *hunting up house members, one by one, teaching them the facts, showing them the rice, etc.,. . .We caught the chief opponent about 6:30* PM. *He listened, asked questions, took all of our material, seemed impressed, but we did not know whether or not we had him convinced. . . . Miss Lacot and I went*

*back at 8:00 PM and stayed until the bill came up. Much to our delight, the last man we talked to, the opposition leader, presented it, said that they had turned it down without knowing the facts. He recited his entire lesson as we taught it to him, showed our charts, showed the rice, and did a wonderful job. Two members fought it in long harangues, but the vote was a resounding "*yes*"! So when the Governor signs it, it becomes a law and Puerto Rico will have the honor of being the first country to pass such a law. We are quite proud.*

The governor signed the bill on 13 May 1951. It required that all rice sold for human consumption must be enriched with thiamin, niacin, and iron. Some years later, Governor Muñoz Marín cited Dr. Roberts's important role in the achievement of rice enrichment for Puerto Rico:

This has been of undoubted benefit to a very extensive portion of the population and Dr. Roberts was one of the major contributors to the program. Often, it was her participation which led directly to various important necessary decisions. To a considerable extent, she was responsible for its success.[6]

Always near the center of operation of the Nutrition Committee, Dr. Roberts tells of one of the committee's encounters with advertisers. The committee wrote letters to sponsors of radio and television programs, approving when the advertising was ethical and calling attention when it was believed not to contribute to public welfare. In Dr. Roberts's words:

There is a malt beverage called Ponche *and the advertising has been terrible,* Ponche *in Puerto Rico means egg-nog. The advertiser says something about that wonderful Ponche [that] mother made with milk, eggs, etc. . . then talks about their Ponche. People get the idea that it contains eggs and milk. Worst of all, they had a program with a clown that children loved. As a part of it, the clown would ask, "What's the best drink in the world?" The children would say "Ponche." It was having a very bad effect on milk drinking. Finally our committee went to see the clown and told him how badly they felt to have him influencing the children that way. He was very nice. He said he thought milk better, but that was what he was paid $12,000 a year to do. But he said that he had two days without a program and he'd do some free advertising for milk those days. He did. Then one day, he came to the girls and said, "My little work for you on the milk cost me my $12,000 job!" Ponche fired him—Then the girls went to see one of the big dairy men. . . and he took over the program! So now the clown asks children, "What is the best drink for children?" And they yell back, "Leche"—Isn't that something?*

It is not surprising that Dr. Roberts should have been drawn into the School Lunch Program shortly after her 1946 arrival in Puerto Rico. Child nutrition was always a high priority for her. In 1947, Maria Socorro Lacot, then supervisor of the School Lunch Program, sought Dr. Roberts's help. Federal funds had become available for the purchase of equipment. She asked for Dr. Roberts's assistance in preparing Puerto Rico's request. As usual, Dr. Roberts's advice was practical. Her proposal was that the lunchroom workers themselves be asked to submit lists of what they needed to prepare meals. The women asked for large spoons, knives, big pots for cooking rice, and buckets to replace cracker tins for carrying water. There were few requests for walk-in freezers, 12-unit ranges, or elaborate storage units.

A serious concern of Dr. Roberts was the quality of dietetic service in hospitals and other institutions in Puerto Rico. She considered improvement a necessity. And when Dr. Roberts held a belief, it was certain that every effort would be made to bring about a change. More trained dietitians were needed. She encouraged students in the Department of Home Economics with an interest in science to major in nutrition and dietetics. Her endeavor met with considerable success. The number of nutrition and dietetics majors increased from five or six in 1943 to 30 in 1950.

A student who graduated from the university with a major in nutrition and dietetics, however, was not yet equipped to be a dietitian. Practical experience in an accredited hospital was an additional requirement of The American Dietetic Association. There was no such program for dietetic training in Puerto Rico. The expense and language difference made an internship on the mainland impossible for most of the students. In 1951, however, the Veterans Administration gave permission for six dietetic graduates to have work experience in the dietary department of their San Patricio Hospital in Río Piedras. Later that same year, The American Dietetic Association officially recognized San Patricio Hospital as a provider of dietetic internship training. The dietetic internship was a joint concern of the Veterans Administration and the San Juan Municipal Hospital, with the University of Puerto Rico serving as coordinator. It was a milestone in providing dietitians for Puerto Rico, and a notable achievement for Dr. Roberts.

Another big step forward for dietetics in Puerto Rico came in 1947, when the Institute for Dietitians was held. The Department of Home Economics arranged for the month-long institute. A consulting dietitian from the United States served throughout the institute, which greatly helped the developing field of dietetics move forward.

Dr. Roberts's wide diversity of community service with the government, the nutrition committee, the dietitians, the Extension Service, and other home economists had a common denominator—making life better for Puerto Rican people.

REFERENCES

1. Roberts LJ: Letter to Thelma A. Dreis, 2 February 1949.
2. Nutrition in the Insular Penitentiary. Report of the committee appointed by Governor Muñoz Marín, 26 February 1951.
3. Roberts LJ, Stefani RL: *Patterns of Living in Puerto Rican Families.* Río Piedras, PR, University of Puerto Rico, 1949.
4. Roberts LJ: Review of Activities in Puerto Rico (from February 1943 to January 1951). Submitted to Chancellor Jaime Benítez, University of Puerto Rico, March 1951.
5. Maretzki A: Where Every Prospect Pleases. Unpublished manuscript, 1978.
6. Muñoz Marín L: Letter to president of Chicago Nutrition Association, 15 September 1956.

CHAPTER 10

Broadening Her Sphere

Lydia Roberts retired for the second time in 1952. Although she retired as head of the Department of Home Economics, she remained a member of the faculty. Many of the ideas for reorganization that she had brought to the department had been accomplished. She did not want to be involved in administrative responsibilities any longer; she preferred teaching and workshops. Looking to the future, she could see a broader scope for Home Economics activities. In her report to Chancellor Jaime Benítez in 1951, she had said:

> *It is our belief that with adequate facilities and support the Department could become one of the most effective agencies for improving the standard of living in Puerto Rico. It could, moreover, serve as a training center for workers from the other Caribbean Islands, and also from the Latin American countries, which have no such program of training. It would thus be rendering a needed service not only in Puerto Rico but over a wider area.*[1]

With such a goal, it is not surprising that, as in her first retirement, Dr. Roberts's activities expanded rather than decreased. Even before retirement they had extended out into the Caribbean. The attention attracted by her workshops seems to have been a factor in the spreading demand for her assistance. It was in 1950, as noted earlier, that she conducted a workshop for a Caribbean group. In 1951 she went to Trinidad to consult with that government regarding programs in home economics and nutrition, and she also represented the United States at a Conference on Nutrition Problems in Latin America that was held in Caracas. Also in 1951, she had a call from the Inter-American Institute of Agricultural Sciences (IAIAS) at Turrialba, Costa Rica, a project of the Organization of American States. The IAIAS wanted Dr. Roberts to plan the development of a home economics program in its Technical Cooperation Program in Latin America. In 1952 she returned to IAIAS. Dr. Ralph H. Allee, director of the institute, asked

Dr. Roberts to make stops on her return to Puerto Rico, in Panama, Colombia, and Venezuela, to take note of their nutrition programs.

At each of these stops, former students took special care of Dr. Roberts—supplementing the plans of the agencies in charge of her visit. There were sights to be seen and special teas and dinners—all of which were thoroughly enjoyed by their former professor and good friend. And Dr. Roberts did not miss the opportunity to let people in those countries know of the nutrition offerings available to them at the University of Puerto Rico.

Dr. Roberts went back to Trinidad in 1952, this time from 30 June to 5 July, to serve as chairman of the Conference on Home Economics and Education in Nutrition. The conference, sponsored by the Caribbean Commission and the Food and Agriculture Organization (FAO) of the United Nations, was attended by 36 delegates and observers from 13 countries, international organizations, and associations. The conference goal was to help interpret the broad scope and purpose of home economics and the contribution it could make to improving living conditions for families and communities.

In 1953 Dr. Roberts was particularly busy with international activities. She was designated by the US Department of State to serve as chairman of the US Delegation to the Third Joint Food and Agriculture Organization/World Health Organization Latin American Nutrition Conference at Caracas. She also represented the United States at a conference on Latin American nutrition problems in Rio de Janeiro. It is probable, however, that the most important activity in Lydia Roberts's eyes was the nutrition training course that she conducted at the University of Puerto Rico. Twenty-six people from the different Caribbean countries attended the course, which was sponsored by the university, the Caribbean Commission, and the Food and Agriculture Organization.

Another international activity in 1953 brought Dr. Roberts to Jamaica for two months to assist with preparations for the introduction of a program in home economics at the newly established University of the West Indies. She was there under the sponsorship of the FAO. In 1954 she returned to Jamaica to assist with course planning, and in 1955 for the inauguration of the program. The inaugural event was attended by the governor, the commissioner of education, and the president of the university. Each made a speech. It was a sufficiently important event to make headlines in the newspaper, with almost a full page of copy. In the summer of 1955, Dr. Roberts was back again, this time to teach courses in the new department.

On Dr. Roberts's return to Puerto Rico, she continued her international activities. She spoke of it as "spending my time in conference." In a short span of time, visitors came from Panama, Brazil, Thailand, Venezuela, England, and

Chile. She commented about them, "It takes a lot of time and telephone calls to plan their schedules, but I learn a lot from them. So, it pays out in the long run."

Near the end of 1955, her international outreach extended as far as Africa—not surprising, perhaps, when one recalls that as a young person she left her home state of Michigan to teach elementary school in Montana.

Dr. Roberts had wanted to go to Africa—and now she was going. It came about in this way: When an FAO representative visited Dr. Roberts in Puerto Rico, she learned of Dr. Roberts's interest in an assignment in an African country. Uganda was requesting the services of a consultant in family living, nutrition, and women's education. Clearly, Dr. Roberts was the person Uganda was asking for. FAO recommended her for the six-week assignment.

A certificate of health was required to qualify for the assignment. When Dr. Roberts consulted her physician, Dr. Ramón M. Suárez, she presented a typical picture of cardiovascular disease; no one could predict when a fatal event might occur. But she wanted so much to go. Withholding medical approval for the trip could hardly be expected to increase her life expectancy. Dr. Suárez signed the health certificate, with the thought that taking the risk was Dr. Roberts's choice.

The purposes of the study in Uganda aligned directly with Dr. Roberts's interests and expertise in seeking attainable solutions to problems. She would observe the work being done to better the standards of living in the homes and she would recommend measures for achieving improvements and ways that FAO could help carry them out. Her letters tell the personal story of the Uganda visit:

> *. . . When I arrived Saturday noon, November 12 [1955] I was taken to the hotel in Entebbe where I spent the night. The next morning I was whisked off by a Community Development Officer (woman). . . to Mbale (pronounce as if Embale) her headquarters. Enroute we had lunch at the beautiful home of a CWO (man) in Jinja. It was a lovely spot overlooking Lake Victoria. Thence we went to a Catholic Mission and spent the night. The next day I was introduced to African women in a big way. Some 85–90 were there. . . Dresses all colors of the rainbow and mixtures of them, singing dancing, etc. I spent 10 days with her and almost every day saw one to two clubs. . . and saw at least 400 women in all not to count at least half that number of men and children hanging around the outside.*

Dr. Roberts was then taken to Kampala, where she visited schools and homes. An African woman, Kisosason Kale, took her on a week-long tour.

> *She is. . . a member of the Legislative Council. She is showing me real African Women's clubs, homes, etc. Yesterday she took me to a club of Nubian women (from the Sudan, originally). . . . About 24 women dressed in*

the gayest clothes you ever dreamed of. . . . They were outdoors cooking their native dishes over hot stones. . . In the evening I was at Mrs. K's home for dinner which was cooked for me especially by three women who came in 10 miles to bring and serve it. It was brought wrapped in layers and layers of banana leaves and was steaming hot.

From Africa, Dr. Roberts went to Rome, where she prepared her report on the Uganda observations. In the report she paid special attention to the Program of Domestic Science in schools and the work with women's clubs in the Department of Community Development. The Departments of Agriculture, Education, and Health were found to contribute significantly to better family living, so attention was also given to their activities.[2]

The purposes set forth for Dr. Roberts's Uganda assignment were fulfilled. Her recommendations were practical and attainable, aimed at the betterment of family living. Her goal of broadening home economics activities had been accomplished. However, there was still work to be done in Puerto Rico.

REFERENCES

1. Roberts LJ: Review of Activities in Puerto Rico (from February 1943 to January 1951). Submitted to Chancellor Jaime Benítez, University of Puerto Rico, March 1951.
2. Roberts LJ: *Report on Home Economics Education and Related Programs in British Protectorate of Uganda.* Rome, Food and Agriculture Organization, 1956.

CHAPTER 11

A Dream Realized

In 1956, the very next day after Dr. Roberts returned to Puerto Rico from the Uganda assignment, Governor Luis Muñoz Marín asked her to have lunch with him and his wife, Inez Mendoza de Muñoz Marín.

> *He wanted to know about Uganda and to find out if I had ideas about what we could do for the lowest income rural families [in Puerto Rico] who hadn't seemed to have been touched by the general economic rise. One thing led to another and finally I had a chance to tell them my "pipedream" of a rural demonstration.*

Dr. Roberts had had the pipedream for a long time. She went on to describe it in her letter:

> *. . . to select a remote rural community of some 100 or so families, make a detailed study of all aspects of living conditions for every family, and then on the basis of the findings have all agencies concerned to plan and carry out a concerted program designed to help raise the standard of living in every family.*
>
> *He fell for it hard, took notes, and said something would come of it. To hasten it, I wrote a tentative plan for it. Whether anything comes of it, is however, doubtful.*

Dr. Roberts was aware of Governor Muñoz Marín's concern for the *jíbaro* (peasant). He had demonstrated this in his support for having dry skim milk on the market at a reasonable price and his crucial actions in bringing about the law requiring the enrichment of rice.

Looking back in the life of Luis Muñoz Marín, it is apparent that even as a young man he concerned himself with social problems. He was well acquainted with the United States. As an adolescent, he had spent some time in Washington, DC, with his father, who was there on matters of Puerto Rican interest. Later, Luis Muñoz Marín was back in the United States on his own, engaged as a writer for the *Nation* and the *American Mercury*. He was a gifted poet and a journalist. In 1931 he returned to Puerto Rico, this time to stay. He entered politics in the Partido Popular Democratico (Popular Democratic Party). The *jíbaro*—a peasant wearing a straw hat—was the symbol of the party; *"Pan, Tierra, Libertad"* (bread, land, liberty) was its slogan. President Roosevelt appointed him governor of Puerto Rico in 1944, the first native Puerto Rican to be appointed to that office. In 1948, by an overwhelming majority, he became the first elected governor of Puerto Rico.[1]

Even though Governor Muñoz Marín was enthusiastic about her dream project, Dr. Roberts held some doubts that anything would come of it. Perhaps she thought of its enormity, the extensive funds that would be needed to carry it out, or maybe that it would simply be too good to be true.

Governor Muñoz Marín was keenly interested in the project, and planned to put his support for it into action at an early date. He expected to call a meeting of the heads of those agencies that would be concerned, to consider the project and, if they approved, to set up a committee to direct it. However, in 1956 Hurricane Santa Ana struck the island. The governor and the heads of agencies focused their attention on the hurricane damage. There was no opportunity for the meeting. Finally, the governor suggested that they wait no longer for him and proceed without him. The responsibility of getting the project under way fell to Dr. Roberts. Governor Muñoz Marín asked the chief of the Budget Bureau to provide the additional funds, but the funding did not provide for the workers' salaries. The employees of the cooperating agencies involved in the project did the work as part of their regular duties. So the only additional funds needed were for the employment of some local workers, for the purchase of a jeep, and for some miscellaneous expenditures. These funds were supplied by the Department of Health.

Early on, the project needed a location that would fill the requirements for a demonstration community. With Esther Seijo de Zayas, then chief of the Bureau of Nutrition of the Department of Health, Dr. Roberts visited suggested locations. Dr. Roberts's evaluation of their choice:

> *It isn't just what we first planned, but in some ways it is better. We wanted a real rural community, and this one is. . . . The school is on the top of a hill with a view in all directions. There are 90 children in the school. They looked so small and undernourished, that we decided we'd take the place. . . and make the project into a nutrition demonstration.*

Doña Elena, in a mountainous region southwest of San Juan, was the community chosen. Although a good road led partway to the town, the last five miles were passable only by jeep, and after a rain, only on foot or on horseback. Approximately 100 families lived in the area in crudely constructed houses, which were small for the size of the family. Two-thirds of the families had more than six members. Tobacco was the chief cultivated crop; it provided only limited amounts of money for food or other necessities.[2]

Since the program at Doña Elena was to be concerned with nutrition primarily, Dr. Roberts thought that the Nutrition Committee might be interested in sponsoring the project. When the proposal was presented to the committee, the vote to do so was unanimous. A subcommittee was made responsible for the direction and operation of the program. It comprised representatives of the Division of Nutrition of the Department of Health, the School Lunch Program of the Department of Public Instruction, the Food Distribution Division of the United States Department of Agriculture, and the Department of Home Economics of the University of Puerto Rico. These and other agencies contributed liberally to the project through the services of their workers and in general support.

The Doña Elena community was not decided upon conclusively until the residents had had an opportunity to learn about the plan and to express their views. The superintendent of schools called a meeting of the people of Doña Elena and explained the plan to them. They were asked to consider whether or not they wished the project to be carried out in their area. The response was decidedly affirmative. "I am sure," one resident said, "that no one in this room, or anyone else, could possibly object to a program like that." He called it a program of the saints. Those present suggested that another meeting be held so that those families not represented also could have the plan explained to them. At the second meeting, those present also welcomed the project and expressed their desire to cooperate. The residents chose people from their community to form a local council that addressed matters of the project.

The program began with home interviews and nutritional checkups of the school children. In the interviews, information relating to the nutrition and food supply of the families was obtained. Since improving the nutritional status of school children was to be the main criterion for judging the success of the program, a check of the children's status before school feeding began was essential. Dr. Roberts's usual approach to a research project was assessment before an experimental program was introduced and evaluation at its conclusion.

As the project got under way, it became clear to the workers in the Doña Elena project that poor nutrition was not the only problem facing this rural community. The community was isolated because the roads were impassable; all the water used in the homes had to be carried by hand; there were no latrines or electricity. The houses needed repair and were too small. Before the end of the first year the program had, of necessity, developed into one for the betterment of all-around living conditions in the home and the community.

A part of Dr. Roberts's dream was "that there should be workers living in the community to carry on the day to day work with the families." Two young people filled those posts in the Doña Elena demonstration community: Carmen Luz Santiago, home economist, and her brother Alejandro Santiago, agronomist. They had grown up in a rural area not far from Doña Elena, and they understood and liked country people. Although both were concerned with all aspects of the program, Carmen was primarily responsible for the school meals and for weighing and measuring the children. She also worked with out-of-school girls and the women. Alejandro was in charge of the home-food-production program. He also was the driver of the jeep and actually became involved in every type of job about the place. "It is due largely to the interest and devoted service of these two workers that the success achieved by the program can be attributed."[2]

Finding a place for Carmen and Alejandro to live was not easy. Dr. Roberts's description of it: ". . . a little house or shack of corrugated tin that was in a terrible condition. . . .We had to 'bulldoze' a road to it as it was in a field with only a foot path. We had to build a latrine, fix windows and doors, replace boards in the floor, etc. Then we gathered together all of the furniture we could find in the University of Puerto Rico storeroom!"

When things were getting under way at Doña Elena, Dr. Roberts wrote Governor Muñoz Marín and told him about it, just enough to "whet his appetite." On receiving her letter, Governor Muñoz Marín invited her to have lunch with him and Mrs. Muñoz Marín, and "to bring Carmen and Alejandro." Dr. Roberts described the encounter:

> *The Governor and Mrs. Muñoz were charmed with my children. They were so pleased that some Puerto Rican young people cared enough for rural people to go and live among them as these two will. The Governor asked me how many other "blind spots" there were in Puerto Rico. I told him that others more familiar with the Island estimated there were 200–300, many much worse than ours. The Governor at once began planning a big project for when we show results of ours, to reach the whole 300! He said the trouble would be to find 300 Carmens and Alejandros to live there! And he was nice enough to add, "And we can't multiply Miss Roberts by 300!"*

Governor Muñoz Marín visited Doña Elena on several occasions. It was, of course, a special event when he did. Dr. Roberts tells of his first visit:

> *I thought that we would go quietly and not tell anybody. But I forgot the security measures for a Governor. When we arrived at Alejandro's place*

(our regular gang), I told him the Governor was coming. His first reaction was one of astonishment, then a look of relief. He then told us that detectives had been at his parents' home the night before asking his parents about him. They were worried for fear he was in some trouble. His mother didn't sleep all night and Alejandro, of course, was wondering what he had done. Hence his relief when he realized the reason for the detective's visit.

The usual gang went up with Alejandro and Mrs. Marchand and waited at "La Casa del Joven" a wayside restaurant near where I told the Governor to come. I had one hour to wait there. The Commissioner of Education arrived an hour early, so we had a full hour to talk to him about educational problems in Puerto Rico and Doña Elena in particular.

The day was sunny and everything perfect. I rode in the jeep with Governor and Mrs. Muñoz. They were good sports. Mrs. Muñoz said she hadn't had so much fun in ages. I told them they were seeing roads at their best *and that was bad enough.*

The Governor was wonderful. He has a gift of talking with the common people and getting them to talk freely to him. So does Mrs. Muñoz. The good part is that their liking and interest are genuine and all recognize it—not just something for political reasons. They visited the school, watched the children eat lunch, then ate the lunch forming a line like children and carrying the trays to the kitchen afterwards. After lunch, we went to the house [of Carmen and Alejandro]. All the local crowd that had assembled followed. They inspected the house, the garden. Then we put all the chairs in the front yard and the people sat and talked with the Governor and Mrs. Muñoz about land, roads, etc. When I said "good bye" to the Governor later, he said, "It was well worth it!" You can imagine how the teachers and workers at Doña Elena, as well as the people, felt and how much good it has done our project. Our trouble is that everyone wants to visit us—all the "big wigs" of the government as well as others. We seem to have started something.

The governor's genuine interest in the welfare of families in isolated rural communities was evidenced by his mentioning Doña Elena in his annual speech to the legislature. He paid special tribute to Dr. Roberts. She said of it,

Imagine being mentioned in a Governor's message! Some Doña Elena people, who have radios, were listening and heard the Governor's speech. They were thrilled to have their tiny barrio *named on such an occasion.*

Governor Muñoz Marín paid a return visit to Doña Elena one and a half years after his first one. As told by Dr. Roberts:

Last Wednesday the Governor went with us up to Doña Elena or rather

we went with him. . . . So a procession of 10 jeeps climbed the road to Doña Elena carrying the Governor, Mrs. Muñoz, Secretary of Agriculture, and top officials, a security man leading the procession. There were some 30 or more persons. All were impressed. From there we drove over a long hard country road to another "pocket"—as the Governor had requested to see another. It was a worse road than Doña Elena. Esther and I rode with the Governor, Alejandro driving. We chuckled to think of all the big-wigs having to bump along behind us because the Governor had told them to come. It was very good for them to see such places, and they were surprised when we told them that according to our preliminary study there are at least 400 such places in Puerto Rico with a population of at least 200,000 people! The place we stopped was a little school in a house. A terrible mess. The woman of the house was a little short, plump person. When she saw the Governor she ran and clasped him around the middle (as far as she could reach) and exclaimed over and over again "El Gobernador, el dueño de Puerto Rico en mi casa!" *[The owner of Puerto Rico in my house!] The Governor was amused.*

The day of the school children's first medical examination was one to be remembered. The events are told best by Dr. Roberts herself.

I wish I could adequately picture our experience at Doña Elena. Dr. Sevringhaus (from the Institute of Nutrition, Columbia University), Dr. Mata (a local pediatrician), my two girls, Carmen Luz and Sylvia, drove in one car, and there were two other loads. Our new red jeep was finally ready for use and it transported us to the place in two trips. The day was satisfactory so far as attendance was concerned and the examinations. The school was full when we arrived. We set up things, and began the examinations, but the doctors could do them only so fast. Imagine a roomful of 150 people, adults and children of all ages, waiting patiently for 5–6 or 7 hours for an examination. . . . We examined 142 in all—pretty good day's work. But the climax came when we had to leave. It rained hard all P.M., *and we knew the road would be practically impassable. We started in the jeep. But it couldn't take us far. We had to get out and walk, and we walked most of the 5 miles to the road, through mud, red clay, sticky and deep puddles of water, over steep hills and down other steep ones with rain coming down much of the time. We slipped and slid the 5 miles in about 3 hours. Dr. Guerra, dental chief of the Health Department, fell 5 times, 3 or 4 of the girls lost their shoes and continued on in stocking feet or barefoot. We were all soaked to the skin and smeared with clay to the knees and on our clothes. You never saw such a sight in your life; I certainly never did. Dr. Sevringhaus and Dr. Mata walked and got smeared like the rest of us. Everyone took it in good spirits, however, and really made a lark out of it. When I got home, I peeled off everything and soaked in a tub of hot water. Then I threw my clothes in and let them soak. My shoes, I think are beyond any further use.*

At the time this letter was written, Dr. Roberts was 79 years old.

Once the assessment had been completed, the next step was planning the improvement program. The basis for it would be the home-interview findings and the physical examinations of the children. Since the emphasis of the project was originally on nutrition, the program for betterment focused on improving the nutrition of the school children and families. The high points of the improvement plan were that the school children would be given three meals a day at school instead of just lunch. The school and lunchroom would be used for teaching and inculcating good food habits. The school children would be weighed weekly and their heights taken monthly, both under standard conditions. Adults would be taught the essentials of good nutrition and how to secure them through everyday foods. Home production of essential foods would be encouraged.

Dr. Roberts felt that parents should know the outcome of the medical examinations of their children, at least in a general way. So a meeting was called on a Sunday afternoon, the time preferred by most families. The meeting was well attended. The findings were shared: the children were not getting all of the nutrients their bodies needed. The "Protective Foods for Puerto Rico" chart outlined the foods needed for good nutrition: milk, protein foods, green and yellow vegetables and fruits, and other fresh fruits. The agronomist explained how the families could produce these foods on their land and added that he would be on hand to help them get their gardens started if they wished.

Those present showed interest in having four more meetings, each one devoted to one of the essential food groups. So the meetings were held on Sunday afternoons, at three-week intervals.

For the meeting on milk, the high-grade milk goat of the university's Department of Home Economics was taken along in the jeep. Word got around that the goat was to be at the meeting, so a large crowd gathered. They watched the milking process and were amazed at the quantity of milk obtained. At this meeting, the government's program for providing cows or milk goats for low-income families was explained. A number of families who could meet the requirements made application.

Dr. Roberts's devotion to her dream can be appreciated when she says, "I go to Doña Elena every Wednesday, leaving here at 6:30 A.M. and also every third Sunday. Between times, I'm trying to tabulate data from the schedules of the families."

The idea of developing other isolated communities after the pattern of Doña

Elena was growing. Governor Muñoz Marín asked Dr. Roberts to work with him in writing a bill requesting $300,000 for such projects. He expected the bill to be passed by the legislature, so he asked Dr. Roberts to attend a conference on plans for the use of the funds. All of this led to her writing, "I feel as if I had started a landslide of some sort and couldn't stop it." The legislature approved the funds. In July 1960, a Commission for the Improvement of Isolated Communities was appointed, and the governor named Dr. Roberts president of the commission. The other members of the commission were Esther Seijo de Zayas of the Department of Health; Margarita Pont Flores of the School Lunch Program; and the Secretaries of Agriculture, Health, Education, and Public Works. The funds appropriated were for building roads, rural electrification, constructing aqueducts, and provided for schools, teacher salaries, and for home economists and agronomists who would work in the areas.

A survey of the isolated rural communities was made. The largest communities and those most in need of improvement were selected for the initiation of the program. The project was necessarily a long-term one, but over a period of years a program similar to the Doña Elena pattern was carried out in each community.

At the end of five years, it was time to evaluate the Doña Elena project. What measurable improvements had there been? There were changes—in the children, their parents, the teachers, the buildings, and grounds. Attendance at school had steadily increased as the program progressed. Eating habits improved. During the first year, the children pushed aside unfamiliar foods and did not eat them. But the proportion of children eating everything on their plates increased until almost 100% of them had "clean plates." This notable success was attributed to regulating portion size to the child and, particularly, to having the teachers eat with the children, with each paying special attention to her own students. The majority of the children showed improved growth in height and weight compared with children in another school without the program, and also according to standard tables for height and weight.

Changes for the better were made in the water supply. From the beginning a major problem of the Doña Elena community was obtaining water for use in the homes. Most of the families carried all the water for household use from some distance. Only a few homes had facilities for catching rain water from the roofs. During the first year of the project, families were encouraged to build eaves on their houses and were helped to find drums to catch the water. At the end of the fifth year, practically all families had eaves and drums. Also, by that time, an aqueduct was well under construction to supply water to three communities, one of which was Doña Elena. When completed, the system would serve 80%

of the Doña Elena families. Hydrants were placed at convenient locations along the road. Those families who could afford it planned to pipe water to their homes. Others would go to the hydrants for it. The group organizer of the Department of Community Education, with the cooperation of the Rural Development Program of the Extension Service at Naranjito, sponsored the water project. It seems safe to propose that such an improvement would happen only in a developing community such as Doña Elena.

None of the homes in the community had electricity at the beginning of this project. At the end of the fifth year, 78% of the families were supplied with it.

For the people of the community, the greatest gain in the five years was improvement of the roads. Two neighboring towns, Comerio and Naranjito, and the Community Education program collaborated in making about half the distance to the school passable by car in any kind of weather. However, several kilometers of the road still remained impassable in rainy weather. So the Commission for the Improvement of Isolated Communities allocated funds for completing the job. Dr. Roberts was still chairman of this commission. By the end of the fifth year a car could go all of the way to the school, whatever the weather. For the people in the community this was a dream come true. Now they could get their products to market and bring needed supplies to the community. It was no longer an isolated community.

An interest in better housing grew steadily during the five years of the project. Encouraged by the increasing interest of families to improve their homes, the Doña Elena sponsors asked the Social Programs Administration to initiate a self-help housing project in the community. The government participated by loaning money to the families for home-building expenses, providing the building materials, and permitting their engineers to direct the construction. The family made a minimum down payment, built the house working cooperatively with other families, and made small monthly payments until the house was paid for.

Originally, over half (54%) of the houses, exclusive of the kitchens, were in a fairly satisfactory condition, and the remaining 46% needed major repairs or needed to be replaced by new ones. Near the end of the third year of the project, 76% of the families were living in houses better in some respects than in 1958. Some families had repaired floors, roofs, or walls; some had built or repaired steps; and many had painted their houses. Some families had added an extra room, either by building on or by dividing space. A few families had built new houses. Near the end of the fifth year, a resurvey showed that approximately 67% of the houses were in good condition; 27%, fair; and only 7%, poor. The improvement in housing indicated the progress being made toward a higher standard of living in the community.

The area around the houses was vastly improved. After five years, it was clean and attractive. Few families had latrines at the beginning; all had them by the fifth year.

Doña Elena, a dream realized. What did it demonstrate? That people, Dr. Roberts's first priority,

> *do not need to be made to realize that they should have such things as better roads, electricity, and a water supply. They merely need to be helped to attain them and encouraged to work together as a community in efforts to do so. . . . But improvements in such matters as food supply for the family, the adequacy of family meals, the care of children, the sanitation and cleanliness of the home and surroundings, and the general standards of living—these must be effected by each individual family.*[2]

After five years of the project, almost all families were living better than before in some respects. Most of them were genuinely interested in doing what they could to make improvements.

Home food production was encouraged and did show some increase over the five years. More vegetable gardens were planted; more fruit trees obtained. The greatest improvement in food animals was the introduction of a better breed of chickens. Some families increased their home milk supply by acquiring high-milk-producing cows through the Dairy Cattle Distribution Program in effect at the time. Many families did not have sufficient land to maintain a cow. Although milk goats might have been a solution, interest in having them had not grown.

Family meals improved in nutritive quality. The greatest change was in the breakfasts. Originally, 70% of the families had only coffee for breakfast; in the last recheck, the number had been reduced to 31%. The other meals were also better. There was increased use of meat, eggs, and milk. The community workers noted that meat consumption increased when electricity was introduced into the area. The small grocery stores were then able to keep fresh meat, and families who could afford it bought it.

The most important change was in the spirit and attitude of the residents of the community. Hope and optimism replaced despair and a feeling that nothing would ever happen to better their lot. "Doña Elena, as the residents will tell you, is not the same place as it was before."[2]

Doña Elena was a research model heretofore unexplored. The model and its architect attracted visitors from around the world. People were the beneficiaries of the Doña Elena project, and for good reason. As Dr. Roberts both proclaimed and demonstrated, "I'm interested . . . in bettering the lot of the common people."[3]

REFERENCES

1. Carrion AM: *Puerto Rico: A Political and Cultural History.* New York, W.W. Norton and Co, 1983.
2. Roberts LJ: *The Doña Elena Project.* Broadview, IL, Photopress, 1963.
3. Roberts LJ: letter to Thelma A. Dreis, 2 February 1949.

CHAPTER 12

Winding Down

The five-year demonstration period of Doña Elena was over in 1961. Dr. Roberts's belief was that the findings of research must be published. The manuscript was ready for publication early in 1962; it did not come off the press until late in 1963. One publisher failed to keep the agreement, another delayed unduly. Not often was a discouraging word ever heard from Dr. Roberts, but regarding this book she said, "I've about given up hope of ever having it printed." But her persistence was worth it. The response to the book pleased her. Not only were there favorable reactions to the publication, but also, as she put it, "flattering comments about yours truly."

The 1963 report of the first five years in Doña Elena marked a milestone for Lydia Roberts. Maybe it was time to slow down a little bit, perhaps even to think of leaving her island, to go "home." After all, she was 84 years old. Her sister, Lillian Roberts, was still living in the apartment on Blackstone Avenue in Chicago; she was 86, and wanted Lydia to come home. Governor Muñoz Marín would not be running for governor again. Dr. Roberts would miss his help and support. Although she never talked much about it herself, she had heart problems. About all she ever said was that she had "had one of her spells." Others were more concerned than she. A doctor friend made a special point to keep an eye on her—to the point that, when Dr. Roberts went to Miami in 1962 to report on the Doña Elena Project at the Annual Meeting of The American Dietetic Association, someone else attending the meeting was charged to keep tabs on Dr. Roberts. Lydia Roberts's thoughts did begin to turn back home—to Chicago and to Michigan, even though it was wrenching to think of leaving Puerto Rico, with its beauty, its wonderful climate, and its warm and friendly people. In her letters to her friend Ethel Austin Martin, she began to ask practical questions. What should she do about her car? She was still driving all of the time in San Juan, but she did not think she would want to drive in Chicago. She would like the car, though, "to run around in Michigan." And in the Blackstone Avenue apartment, there still were notes and card files on the child growth and food intake data. She and her friend and former student, Bernice Wait Wood, had been considering getting that material ready for publication.

While Dr. Roberts pondered these questions, however, there was still much to be done in Puerto Rico. Nineteen sixty-three and the first part of 1964 flew by. Sometime in mid-1964 she gave up the apartment in Santurce, gave away the desk and chest with which she had supplemented the hotel furniture, and returned to Chicago. This time, in addition to their usual visits with family and friends, she and her sister apparently spent some time looking at retirement communities and considering possible changes in their living arrangements. The result? Dr. Roberts wrote her friends in Puerto Rico to see if they could get her apartment back—she wasn't ready to leave yet!

Fortunately, she was able to get the same apartment in Santurce again, although "they put in new furniture. . . and so said they had to raise the rent. I preferred the old!" Replacements were found for the desk and chest—inexpensive ones, because "I didn't want to invest much in them for a few months use and I have a feeling this is my last year really living here, though I'll probably always want to come back for brief stays." She was obviously glad to be back. The weather was lovely—"I feel a hundred percent better than in Chicago," she wrote. Lil came for her usual winter visit in February. There were social and professional activities. She was back at work in her office at the university, and the nutrition textbook for Puerto Rico was taking form. With a little more time to work on it, she told friends that she actually had hopes it would be finished soon. Not that she could work on it full time—there was a constant stream of visitors and many requests for help and consultation.

Many of the visitors came expressly to see Doña Elena and to learn about community-development techniques that had come out of that project. Those techniques were used in nutrition projects in many other parts of the world—Doña Elena was, perhaps, one of the best teaching devices Dr. Roberts had ever developed.

So, although she still thought about going home and, although she knew her work would be in good hands if she left, she was glad to be back in Puerto Rico and still busy in 1965.

On 28 May 1965, it ended.

Those gathered at the funeral home in Puerto Rico on 29 May did not want to believe it. Lillian Roberts was there to receive them—those from government, the university, the rural area, the community. Dr. Roberts had worked with all of them to better the life of the people of Puerto Rico. But now they were to go it alone, leaning on the heritage she had left them.

Dr. Roberts's remains were returned to Martin for burial in the family plot. "We could not send her body to the States alone to be buried without her friends from Puerto Rico attending the funeral," one of her associates wrote. "So we all pitched in and paid Elizabeth Sánchez's trip [accompanying Lillian Roberts] to Martin, Michigan, with instructions to buy the prettiest flowers for the funeral from the many friends she left in Puerto Rico."

CHAPTER 13

The Test of Time

Lydia Roberts's life ended in Puerto Rico in 1965, but her work went on. On a visit to Puerto Rico by one of the authors in 1986, her name and her influence were found to be still very much alive.

Dr. Roberts did a good job of preparing for the future of the Department of Home Economics and especially of the nutrition programs in Puerto Rico. A strong foundation lay beneath the structures she had helped erect. Perhaps the most important legacy Lydia Roberts left to "her island" was a group of dedicated and inspired people who were also a well-trained work force fully capable of carrying on without her. This was "the gang," as she called them in her letters.

In developing the Department of Home Economics at the University of Puerto Rico, Dr. Roberts had emphasized good training. Faculty members and graduates of the department were encouraged to go to the mainland to work on advanced degrees. When they returned to Puerto Rico, most of them found it possible to combine a professional career with marriage and a family. By this time Dr. Roberts apparently had given up any idea she might have had that the two were not compatible! Indeed, she loved being surrounded by these young people and their families. And they loved her, as this 1986 comment attests:

> *To many members of the Home Economics faculty at the University of Puerto Rico she was like a beloved aunt. She would involve you in one project after the other, pushing you and forcing you to grow under her guidance. Some of the younger (less reverent) faculty referred to her as "la Titi" [auntie] and included her in family outings to El Yunque, to the beach and to our homes. . . . When she died we mourned her as family.*

In 1965 members of "the gang" were ready and able to proceed on their own. Their sense of loss was acute, but they had learned from Dr. Roberts not to dwell in the past, but to look to the future.

Their first task was to notify Dr. Roberts's many friends of her death. A black-bordered note was sent out:

> *Her friends in Puerto Rico regret to inform you that our beloved Dr. Lydia Jane Roberts passed away suddenly, Friday, May 28 at Río Piedras, Puerto Rico.*
>
> *Her sister, Lillian, came to Puerto Rico to accompany her remains to Martin, Michigan, where burial took place Monday, May 31, 1965. The staff of the Home Economics Department of the University of Puerto Rico, members of the Puerto Rico Dietetic Association, Nutrition Committee, and Home Economics Association, students and other friends will forever remember her for her contribution, guidance, inspiration, and her love for Puerto Rico.*[1]

Her desk and office were cleared, and one room in the quarters of the Home Economics Department was dedicated to her memory. Her books and papers were placed there for others to use, and the room would provide work and study space for students. The Sala Roberts (Roberts Room) was dedicated 7 June 1966 with the unveiling of a bust of Dr. Roberts by Puerto Rican sculptor José Buscaglia. On one wall of the room is a large bronze plaque inscribed with a quotation from University of Puerto Rico President Jaime Benítez's commencement address of 4 June 1965, which praised Dr. Roberts's work at the university. This memorial was important to her associates in the Home Economics Department of the university.

Dr. Roberts herself, through a bequest to The American Dietetic Association for a fellowship in the field of public health nutrition, had provided aid for future nutritionists interested in working directly with people. However, her many friends felt that there should be another, larger, memorial as well, one that would reflect the broader aspects of her work in Puerto Rico, the United States, and abroad. A committee was appointed to consider the possibilities. It was the consensus of the committee, and of others they consulted, that "there is no better way to accomplish this than by creation of an endowment fund that will support a lectureship to be known as the Lydia J. Roberts Memorial Lecture to be delivered once a year at the University of Puerto Rico by a noted teacher or investigator in nutrition, home economics, or related fields."[2] A letter was sent out to announce this decision and to request contributions to the memorial fund.

The response was immediate and gratifying. Contributions came in from old friends, former students, professional associates, professional organizations, business concerns, and international agencies. By the time of the first lecture, in 1966, the fund had reached more than $10,000. Further contributions as well as interest on the principal have kept the lectureship fund going.

The first lecture was held on 31 October 1966, with Dr. William J. Darby of Vanderbilt University as the speaker. On the speakers' platform were Jaime Benítez, president of the University of Puerto Rico, who spoke on the inauguration of the lectureship; Ruth Davila Fogleman, chairman of the Memorial Lecture Committee, and Ethel Austin Martin, longtime close friend of Dr. Roberts, who told some of the outstanding features of Lydia Roberts's life. Dr. Conrado Asenjo of the University of Puerto Rico School of Medicine introduced Dr. Darby, who spoke on "Nutritional Problems of International Importance," including some consideration of the world food supply and population. On the afternoon of the following day Dr. Darby gave a second lecture on "Approaches to the Estimation of Nutritional Requirements of the Human Being." The same pattern of two lectures, one in the evening and one on the following afternoon, has continued through the years.

There have been, of course, many changes in Puerto Rico since Lydia Roberts's death. San Juan, still the population center of the island, has had tremendous growth. Urban sprawl has engulfed nearby communities, and a network of freeways is crowded with commuter traffic. Modern buildings and shopping malls are monuments to progress. Despite these changes, the city still retains evidence of and pride in its Spanish heritage.

Along with the city of San Juan, the University of Puerto Rico also has grown. In 1986 there were nearly 19,000 students on the Río Piedras campus. The Department of Home Economics became the School of Home Economics in 1964, shortly before Dr. Roberts's death. A graduate program in home economics was initiated in 1972. In 1946, when Dr. Roberts became head of the department, there were only about 50 majors; in 1986 there were approximately 500 students in the School of Home Economics. Five undergraduate programs are offered, but by far the largest number of students choose to enroll in nutrition and dietetics. Three dietetic internships approved by The American Dietetic Association are now available on the island.[3]

Many of the changes in the Department of Home Economics probably would have come about in the normal course of events, but the influence of Lydia Roberts is still strong. A number of the current staff members who were students or young faculty in Dr. Roberts's day remember her vividly. Present-day students know about her through the sign outside Room 202 that proclaims it the "Sala Roberts." The Sala Roberts is a room of which Dr. Roberts would approve. It contains a sizable collection of books and periodicals, and, most important, the department's audiovisual equipment has its home there. Overhead projectors and slide projectors are available. An assistant is on hand to check out the equipment and to instruct in its use. Classes often come for demonstrations on the use of the equipment or for instruction on the preparation of visual aids. Perhaps there are still felt-tipped markers and wrapping paper on hand! There is nearly always a group of students using the room for work or study. The remaining personal files of Lydia Roberts are still available in a small adjoining room.

The Nutrition Committee has remained active. In 1970 the committee issued a statement listing the activities in which it had been engaged since the first workshop held in 1943 under Dr. Roberts's direction:

> *. . . many socio-economic, health and nutritional changes have occurred in Puerto Rico. . . new programs have been initiated, and new problems constantly emerge as a result of the dramatic change which the island is undergoing. In view of this situation, we feel the urgent need to evaluate what has been done to date and what priorities should be assigned for the future, based on our real present and projected needs for the next decade.*[4]

A workshop for the evaluation of food and nutrition programs in Puerto Rico was held in April 1970. In the course of the workshop, information was gathered for updating applied-nutrition programs such as food distribution, school lunch, and breakfast centers "within the context of the new advances in nutrition and food technology, and in socio-economic conditions that have taken place during the last twenty-six years."[4] The workshop produced an extensive list of detailed recommendations.[5]

Dr. Roberts's pipedream, which had led to the demonstration at Doña Elena, has not been forgotten, either. The Commission for the Improvement of Isolated Communities still exists, even though few, if any, communities really meet that description any more.

In 1983 Doña Elena was the site of a second research study, "Doña Elena Twenty-Seven Years Later," carried out by a Puerto Rican graduate student working on her doctorate at Columbia University.[6] Workers on the 1983 project found conditions much different from those encountered in 1958. Doña Elena could be reached in about an hour's drive from San Juan. Freeway traffic, not muddy roads, slows the trip now. The beautiful mountain scenery, with San Juan barely visible in the distance, has not changed, but paved roads crisscross the area, and modern houses with pretty gardens are the rule. Members of the recent research team (along with many current residents, no doubt) must have found it difficult to believe that 27 years earlier the road to Doña Elena had been impassable at times.

Members of "the gang" remember it vividly, however. All of them recall many hazardous journeys by jeep or truck, and all of them still talk about the famous walk down the mountain on the day of the first physical examinations of the children. Dr. Roberts's description of it in her letter (see chapter 11) is rather restrained in comparison to their recollections. "It took three hours and forty minutes to get to the main road," said one. "I know. I timed it." Nearly everybody—and apparently quite a group made the trek—lost their shoes, and several of them fell. In fact, one of the pediatricians, Dr. Mata, broke his arm in a fall. Dr. Roberts fell, too, and was carried part of the way by Carmen and Alejandro Santiago. But, despite the difficulties, none seemed to regard it as more than just another exciting day in the history of the work at Doña Elena.

Dr. Roberts certainly has not been forgotten in Doña Elena. Just the mention of her name brings smiles to the faces of people who lived there at the time of the project. Among the community leaders at that time were the Díaz family—Don Pablito, his wife Doña Conchita, and their children—who still live in Doña Elena. According to project workers, the Diaz house was typical of most of those in the town—a rough wooden shack. It is still typical of most houses in the community, but with a difference. Today Mr. and Mrs. Díaz live in an attractive cement-block house surrounded by a beautiful garden. Inside, comfortable furniture reflects the family's increased prosperity. The kitchen would be any cook's joy. The walls and counters are ceramic tile in a soft shade of green, a color repeated in the appliances. A side-by-side refrigerator and freezer, an electric stove, and a stainless-steel sink are all spotlessly clean and well kept. The Díazes' married daughter and her family live next door in another attractive house. The daughter drives to Bayamon, a nearby town, to her job as a dietary technician at the government hospital. She says her interest in this kind of work stems from the days of the Doña Elena project, when she was just a little girl who was much impressed with all the workers who came to their village, especially Dr. Roberts.

Lydia Roberts's name is still familiar in Doña Elena, even to newcomers, for the town community center was named in her honor. In recent years the Centro Communal Dra. Roberts (Dr. Roberts Community Center) has served as headquarters for a Headstart Project. The children appear healthy and happy looking, alert and full of energy, a fitting tribute to the work started 27 years earlier.

The "gang" of whom Dr. Roberts wrote so often was still largely intact in 1986. Most were still professionally active. A few had reached retirement age, and a few had left professional life for personal reasons. Several were members of the university faculty. One was director of the home economics portion of the Isolated Community program. Another was director of nutrition services at the School of Medicine. Others held a variety of nutrition-related positions.

Members of the group remain good friends—the kind of friendship that comes from having shared a stimulating experience. They all speak of Dr. Roberts with love and affection. "We were young, and so excited about what we were doing. Working with her was a wonderful experience. She taught us to do our best," said one. "I think of her every day," said another. "Whenever I plan a new project, I think, 'Now what would Dr. Roberts do?'" Another person said, "I think perhaps we saw her in a different way than her students in the United States did. When she was here, especially after she gave up the headship, she was no longer bound by professional ties. She could be herself, let herself go."

On the occasion of the fifth Lydia J. Roberts Memorial Lecture, in 1970, Dr. H. Ellis Plyler, a member of the University of Puerto Rico Department of Education, gave the closing remarks. He conveyed, in an effective way, what it was that made Dr. Roberts different, made her a force for human betterment in Puerto Rico. *Needs,* he said, dictate people's efforts to earn a living, support a family, or maintain status. But *possibilities* may also influence the decisions of their lives:

> *Dr. Roberts was one who gave her life over to the possibilities. She had a stable, effective satisfying life. . . . But she came to Puerto Rico with the possibility that her experience and knowledge could bring a more abundant life for the families of Puerto Rico. She could have said "I'm too old. I've done my share. Let me enjoy my retirement in peace." But she took the risk of possibility. She rode in a jeep over country lanes, crossing rivers without bridges; walked through mud and swamp to visit the most isolated families; she made friends, she made enemies; she argued, cajoled and insisted, but always giving herself to the dream of a better life for Puerto Rican families.*[7]

Because of her willingness to risk the possibilities, others came to share the dream, and still work to make the dream come true.

REFERENCES

1. Note from Lydia J. Roberts file, Sala Roberts. School of Home Economics, University of Puerto Rico, Río Piedras.
2. Letter sent out announcing Lydia J. Roberts Memorial Lectures. From Lydia J. Roberts file, School of Home Economics, University of Puerto Rico, Río Piedras.
3. Colón de Reguero L: *La Escuela de Economía Doméstica de la Universidad de P.R.* Río Piedras, PR, School of Home Economics, University of Puerto Rico, 1982.
4. Proposal for the evaluation of food and nutrition programs in Puerto Rico. San Juan, Nutrition Committee of Puerto Rico, 1970.
5. Final Recommendations, Interagency Food and Nutrition Workshop, April 1970. San Juan, Nutrition Committee of Puerto Rico, 1970.
6. Vincens de Sánchez L: Dona Elena Twenty-Seven Years Later. DEd thesis. New York, Columbia University, 1986.
7. Plyler HE: Closing remarks, Lydia J. Roberts Memorial Lecture, 1970. From Lydia J. Roberts file, Sala Roberts, School of Home Economics, University of Puerto Rico, Río Piedras.

EPILOGUE

From what we know of Lydia Roberts, it is unlikely that she spent much time thinking of her past accomplishments—there were too many things to plan for in the future. Even the last morning of her life was that way—she never ran out of things to do. If she *had* taken time to think back over her life, she probably would have considered herself a very fortunate woman—fortunate in her abilities, fortunate that she was able to develop those abilities through education and training, fortunate that she had been in the right places at the right times to make the most of her abilities and training.

Lydia Roberts finished high school just as educational and professional opportunities for women were beginning to open up. Her family apparently did not feel that she should stay in Martin and be a homebody, but encouraged her in her desire for education and a career. She came onto the nutrition stage just as the curtains were opening on a new and exciting professional field, in which she would eventually play a starring role. She was a member of the faculty of the Department of Home Economics of the University of Chicago at a time when it was making major contributions in the field. As the importance of the department waned, her time was increasingly filled with commitments at the national level. When retirement came, new tasks awaited her—and certainly if anyone was ever in the right place at the right time, it was Lydia Roberts in Puerto Rico between 1945 and 1965. Not only was there a need for the kind of changes she would bring about, but Governor Muñoz Marín's concern for the *jíbaro* and Chancellor Jaime Benítez's concern for changing educational patterns gave her almost unprecedented opportunities. It almost seemed that all Dr. Roberts had to do was to speak, and funds and support were at hand. Obviously, this reaction really came as a result of her hard and productive work—but after her first few years in Puerto Rico, Dr. Roberts had little or no difficulty in selling her ideas to these two men.

If Lydia Roberts had lived longer, the atmosphere might have been somewhat different. Governor Muñoz Marín left office in 1964, and many changes took place in Puerto Rico. Dr. Roberts had established her programs firmly, however, and they were still working well several years after her death. It is likely that she simply would have moved on to other new and interesting tasks.

Certainly Dr. Roberts's accomplishments were great—but if this account of them makes her sound like a paragon of virtue, we should quickly point out that she was very much a human being, not a saint. Although most of her students and associates were enthusiastic in their evaluations, there were probably few who had not at some time felt the cutting edge of her disapproval—she never did have much tolerance for procrastination. And some never penetrated the outer layer of her reserve, never felt at ease with her—nor she with them.

If Lydia Roberts had looked back on her career she probably would have pointed out that she never made any major discovery in nutrition science—no great breakthrough came about as the result of her work. But she could look with pride at the contribution of a solid body of information, particularly in the field of child nutrition, and to the practical application of nutrition science to the everyday problems of human existence. In this she was unexcelled. Life is better for many people in the world today thanks to Lydia Roberts's influence. Whether these changes came about because of her direct influence, or indirectly, as a result of her teaching and "spreading the nutritional gospel," is immaterial.

In writing this biography we have tried to present the many accomplishments of a remarkable woman, as seen through the eyes of her students, her associates, and those who benefited from the changes she brought about. It all comes down to this:

Thank you, Dr. Roberts. *Muchas gracias, Doctora.*

APPENDIX 1
Published Works

This listing of publications and statements concerning them is from an article by Ethel Austin Martin, titled "The Life Works of Lydia J. Roberts," published in the *Journal of The American Dietetic Association* (49:199–302, 1966).

BOOKS

Dr. Roberts's . . . books represent three broad interests in her professional life: (a) the field of nutrition education for children, in which she was a pioneer in research, teaching, and writing; (b) her belief in the need for relating the university curriculum in home economics to patterns of living in the community; and (c) her deep concern for improving the nutritional welfare of low-income families.

Nutrition Work With Children. Chicago: Univ. of Chicago Press, 1927; revised, 1935.

Patterns of Living in Puerto Rican Families (with Stefani, R. L.). Río Piedras, P.R.: Univ. of Puerto Rico, 1949.

The Doña Elena Project—A Better Living Program in an Isolated Rural Community. Río Piedras, P.R.: Univ. of Puerto Rico Book Store, 1963.

REPORTS OF RESEARCH AND EXPERIMENTAL PROGRAMS

At the University of Chicago, Dr. Roberts supervised the nutrition research of students working for master's and doctoral degrees in the Department of Home Economics. The theses which resulted were, in turn, adapted to reports published in professional journals, many of which appeared with the student investigators as co-authors. In such cases, the names of the collaborators are indicated. . . . A glance at the list suggests the remarkable variety of both laboratory and community studies which have contributed to nutritional knowledge.

A cheap homemade soy-bean meal for diabetics (with Miller, E. W.). *J. Home Econ.* 10:64, 1918.

A malnutrition clinic as a university problem in applied dietetics. *J. Home Econ.* 11:95, 1919.

A dietary study made in a day nursery by the individual method (with Waite, M.). *J. Home Econ.* 17:80, 142, 1925.

A nutrition study on an Indian reservation (with Stene, J. A.). *J. Am. Dietet. A.* 3:215, 1928.

Results of dietary and hygienic control of ten non-gaining preventorium children (with Hord, N.). *J. Am. Dietet. A.* 4:77, 1928.

Overcoming food dislikes. A study with evaporated milk (with Hollinger, M.). *J. Home Econ.* 21:923, 1929.

Studies in the food requirement of adolescent girls (with Wait, B.). 1. The energy intake of well-nourished girls 10 to 16 years of age. 2. Daily variations in the energy intake of the individual. 3. The protein intake of well-nourished girls 10 to 16 years of age. 4. The mineral intake of 38 well-nourished girls 10 to 16 years of age. *J. Am. Dietet. A.* 8:209, 323, 1932; 8:403, 1933; 9:124, 1933.

The supplementary value of dry skim milk in institution diets (with Carlson, L., and MacNair, V.). *J. Am. Dietet. A.* 10:317, 1934.

A clinical comparison of the antirachitic value of irradiated yeast and of cod liver oil (with Compere, E. L., and Porter, T. E.). *Am. J. Dis. Child.* 50:55, 1935.

Hemoglobin and red cell content of the blood of normal women during successive menstrual cycles (with Leverton, R. M.). *J.A.M.A.* 106:1459, 1936.

Seasonal variations in capillary resistance of institution children (with Blair, R., and Bailey, M.). *J. Pediat.* 11:626, 1937.

The iron metabolism of normal young women during consecutive menstrual cycles (with Leverton, R. M.). *J. Nutr.* 13:65, 1937.

Effect of a milk supplement on the physical status of institutional children. 1. Growth in height and in weight (with Blair, R., Lenning, B., and Scott, M.). 2. Ossification of the bones of the wrist (with MacNair, V.). 3. Progress of dental caries (with Englebrecht, S., Blair, R., Williams, W., and Scott, M.). *Am. J. Dis. Child.* 56:287, 494, 805, 1938.

Vitamin A in the blood of normal adults. The effect of a depletion diet on blood values and biophotometer readings (with Steininger, G., and Brenner, S.). *J.A.M.A.* 113:2381, 1939.

Effect of dietary supplement on ossification of the bones of the wrist in institutional children. 2. Effect of a cod liver oil supplement (with MacNair, V.). *Am. J. Dis. Child.* 58:295, 1939).

The supplementary value of the banana in institution diets. 1. Effect on growth in height and weight, ossification of the carpals, and changes in Franzen indices (with Blair, R., Austin, G., and Steininger, G.). 2. Capillary resistance and reduced ascorbic acid in the blood plasma (with Brookes, M. H., Blair, R., Austin, G., and Noble, I.). *J. Pediat.* 15:25, 43, 1939.

Biophotometer test as index of nutritional status for vitamin A (with Steininger, G.). *Arch. Int. Med.* 64:1170, 1939.

A study of the ascorbic acid requirements of children of early school age (with Roberts, V.). *J. Nutr.* 24:25, 1942; *Fed. Proc.* 1:191, 1942.

Dark adaptation of children in relation to dietary levels of vitamin A (with Oldham, H., MacLennan, K., and Schultz, F. W.). *J. Pediat.* 20:740, 1942; *J. Nutr.* 21:7 (No. 6, Suppl. 7), 1941.

The iron requirement of children of the early school age (with Johnston, F. A.). *J. Nutr.* 23:181, 1942.

The relation of liver stores to the occurrence of early signs of vitamin A deficiency in the white rat (with Brenner, S., and Brookes, M. C. H.). *J. Nutr.* 23:459, 1942.

The ascorbic acid requirements of school-age girls (with Roberts, V. M., Brookes, M. H., Koch, P., and Shelby, P.). *J. Nutr.* 26:539, 1943.

Effects of vitamin A depletion in young adults (with Brenner, S.). *Arch. Int. Med.* 71:474, 1943; *Fed. Proc.* 1:188, 1942.

Results of providing a liberally adequate diet to children in an institution. 1. Acceptance of foods and changes in the adequacy of diets consumed (with Blair, R., and Greider, M.). 2. Growth in weight and height (with Blair, R., and Greider, M.). 3. Blood and urinary excretion studies before and after dietary improvement (with Oldham, H., and Young, M.). *J. Pediat.* 27:393, 410, 418, 1945.

Riboflavin excretions of young women on diets containing varying levels of the B vitamins (with Davis, M. V., and Oldham, H. G.). *J. Nutr.* 32:143, 1946.

Thiamin excretions and blood levels of young women on diets containing varying levels of the B vitamins, with some observations on niacin and pantothenic acid (with Oldham, H. G., and Davis, M. V.). *J. Nutr.* 32:163, 1946.

INTERPRETIVE ARTICLES—APPLICATION OF NUTRITIONAL PRINCIPLES

As a result of her research and her wide professional experience, Dr. Roberts was frequently invited by related professional groups to present to them concepts of nutrition education with which they wished to become acquainted. Often these interpretive talks were later published in the professional journals of the organizations before which she spoke. The following list includes such articles, as well as others prepared specifically for publication.

Review of some recent literature on malnutrition in children. *J. Home Econ.* 11:5, 1919.

Malnutrition, the school's problem. *Elementary School J.* 22:457, 1922.

The nutrition specialist in the health program (read in abstract before the Am. Child Health Assn., Detroit, October, 1923). *Hosp. Social Serv.* 9:245, 1924.

Weight as a measure of nutrition. *J. Home Econ.* 16:455, 1924.

Teaching children to like wholesome foods (read in abstract before the Am. Public Health Assn., Detroit, Oct. 22, 1924.). *Amer. J. Public Health* 15:52, 1925.

The prevalence of non-hunger among children and some of its contributing factors (presented at the Northwest Conf. on Child Health and Parent Education). Minneapolis: Univ. of Minn. Press, 1927, p. 54.

The place of nutrition in the school program. *The Commonwealth* (Mass. Dept. Public Health) 15:77 (Oct., Nov., Dec.), 1928.

How a teacher can judge the nutrition of school children. *Elementary School J.* 29:189, 1928.

The dietitian and normal nutrition. *J. Am. Dietet. A.* 5:11, 1929.

The psychologists study eating habits. *Child Study* 7:35 (Nov.), 1929.

The dietitian in social service (presented before The Am. Dietet. Assn., Detroit, Oct. 9, 1929). *J. Am. Dietet. A.* 5:286, 1930.

Food selection for children. *Child Health Bull.* 6:3 (Jan.), 1930.

Nutrition needs of the school child and the responsibility of the home economics teacher. *J. Home Econ.* 24:961, 1932.

The energy requirements of children after infancy (with Wait, B., unsigned). In *Nutrition,* Pt. III of Growth and Development of the Child. White House Conf. on Child Health and Protection. Sect. I, Medical Service. N.Y.: Century Co., 1932.

Coffee, tea, and cocoa for children (with Hawks, J., unsigned). In *Nutrition,* Pt. III of Growth and Development of the Child. White House Conf. on Child Health and Protection. Sect. I, Medical Service. N.Y.: Century Co., 1932.

Home Economics—Vocations for Those Interested in It. Vocational Series No. 1. Chicago: Bd. of Vocational Guidance & Placement. Univ. of Chicago, 1932.

The home economics teacher and the school health program. *J. Mich. School Masters Club* 35:201, 1933.

Scientific feeding of children. *J. Amer. Dent. Assn.* 21:44, 1934.

The school lunch as a health agency. *Hygeia* 12:753, 1934.

Is home economics research meeting its challenge? *J. Home Econ.* 29:677, 1937.

Diet is an important factor in the prevention and control of dental caries. *Nutr. News* 1:5 (Dec.), 1937.

Fortification in a general program for better nutrition. *Milbank Mem. Fund Quart.* 17:230, 1939.

Status of nutrition work with children. *Ann. Am. Acad. Political and Social Sci.* 212:111, 1940.

Practical methods for assessing nutritional status. *J. Health Phys. Ed* 12:226, 1941.

A teacher-education project in improving child nutrition (with Blair, R.). *School Life* 26:273, 1941.

Scientific basis for the Recommended Dietary Allowances. *N. Y. J. Med.* 44:59, 1944.

Present day concepts of nutritional requirements. *Proc Inst. Med. Chicago* 15:22, 1944.

Improvement of the nutritional status of American people. *J. Home Econ.* 36:401, 1944.

Home economics education and related programs in Uganda. Rome: Food & Agric. Org., 1956 (mimeo).

Beginnings of the Recommended Dietary Allowances (presented before The Am. Dietet. Assn., Miami, Oct. 25, 1958). *J. Am. Dietet. A.* 34:903, 1958.

GOVERNMENT BULLETINS

Dr. Roberts was commissioned to develop five government bulletins during her professional life. The second, third, and fourth bulletins on the following list were outcomes of her own and collaborative research in the areas indicated by the respective titles. The remaining bulletins—first and last on the list—present, respectively, an analysis of the understanding of malnutrition in children in 1919 and a positive program for nutritional guidance of children more than two decades later.

What Is Malnutrition? U.S. Children's Bureau Pub. No. 59, 1919; revised, 1927.

The Nutrition and Care of Children in a Mountain County of Kentucky. U.S. Children's Bureau Pub. No. 110, 1922.

Children of Preschool Age in Gary, Indiana. Pt. II. Diet of the Children. U.S. Children's Bureau Pub. No. 122, 1922.

The Child Health School. Conducted in the School of Education of the University of Chicago, Summer, 1920. U.S. Bureau of Education School Health Studies No. 2, 1923.

The Road to Good Nutrition (in collaboration with members of the Children's Bureau staff). U.S. Children's Bureau Pub. No. 270, 1942; revised, 1947.

POPULAR AND SEMI-POPULAR MATERIALS

The items immediately following comprise a sampling of the many materials which Dr. Roberts prepared to help professional colleagues simplify and dramatize nutrition for the lay public. Included are a few tools, such as the food models, which she developed primarily for teaching children.

Why drink milk? *Mother and Child* 3:548, 1922.

From Danger Valley to Safety Hill (health play for children). Private publication, 1923.

Teaching children to eat wholesome foods. *Hygeia* 2:135, 1924.

Food Models (book of outline drawings of fifty foods, life-size—the first food models available). Private publication, 1924.

Cutting down on candy. *Hygeia* 2:411, 1924.

Food in Relation to a Strong Body and Sound Teeth (with Wightman, G. S., and Boggess, B.). Educational Health Circ. No. 23. Springfield, Ill.: Dept. of Public Health, 1927.

The Cost of an Adequate Diet. Chicago: Dept. of Home Econ., Univ. of Chicago, 1928.

Teaching health through the school lunch. *Normal Instructor & Primary Plans.* Oct., 1930, p. 44.

Teaching children to drink milk. *Normal Instructor & Primary Plans,* Nov., 1930, p. 65.

Teaching children to eat fruit regularly. *Normal Instructor & Primary Plans,* Dec., 1930, p. 60.

Sleep for school children. *Normal Instructor & Primary Plans,* Jan., 1931, p. 58.

Teaching children to eat good breakfasts. *Normal Instructor & Primary Plans,* Feb., 1931, p. 70.

Teaching the place of sweets in the diet. *Normal Instructor & Primary Plans,* March, 1931, p. 56.

Teaching children to eat vegetables. *Normal Instructor & Primary Plans,* April, 1931, p. 54.

Steps in the production of clean, safe milk. *Normal Instructor & Primary Plans,* May, 1931, p. 60.

How the housewife spends her food dollar. *Natl. Mag. of Home Econ. Student Clubs* 6:17 (Feb.), 1942.

Off to a good start with proper foods. *Nation's Schools* 29:34 (June), 1942.

PUBLICATIONS BASED ON RESEARCH AND PROGRAMS IN PUERTO RICO

Dr. Roberts spent the final twenty years of her life at the University of Puerto Rico, where she wrote of nutrition and nutrition education on the island. Much of the material reflects her own research and the programs she directed or sponsored. Some of the publications, as indicated on the list, were joint efforts with others. A number of articles were written in English and appeared in journals on the mainland. These are in the first segment of the list. They are followed by bulletins and articles in Spanish issued by agencies in Puerto Rico.

In English

The Puerto Rico Workshop. Presented before Interdepartmental Nutrition Committee, Washington, D.C., July 15, 1943. Mimeo, 1943.

Nutrition in Puerto Rico. *J. Am. Dietet. A.* 20:298, 1944.

Patterns of Living in Puerto Rican Families (see list of books).

Home economics in Puerto Rico. *J. Home Econ.* 41:552, 1949.

A practical nutrition program for Puerto Rico. *Nutr. Rev.* 8:321, 1950.

Food for Your Family. San Juan, P.R.: P.R. Dept. of Education, 1952 (trans. from Spanish by Caribbean Commission).

Some hints on how to have a successful meeting. Río Piedras, P.R.: Univ. of Puerto Rico, 1952 (mimeo).

Caribbean Conference on Home Economics and Nutrition. Dept. of State Bull. No. 27. Río Piedras, P.R.: Univ. of Puerto Rico, 1952.

A basic food pattern for Puerto Rico. *J. Am. Dietet. A.* 30:1097, 1954.

Acerola—miracle of the Caribbean. *Am. J. Nursing* 57:1148, 1957.

The Doña Elena Project (see list of books).

Developing a home economics program to serve the needs of a country—a case example in Puerto Rico. Presented at a conference of Land Grant College Home Economics Units, concerned with the cooperative development of home economics in other countries, June 5, 1963. Stillwater: Okla. State Univ., 1963 (mimeo).

A nutrition survey of three rural Puerto Rican communities (with Plough, I.C., Fernández-López, N. A., and Angel, C. R.). *Bol. Assoc Med. P. Rico* 55:1 Dec. Suppl., 1963.

A cooperative nutrition research program for Puerto Rico. 1. Background and general plan. 2. Nutritional status of the population. Clinical and laboratory examinations (with Plough, I. C., Fernández, N. A., and Angel, C. R.). *J. Am. Dietet. A.* 44:18,22, 1964.

Nutritional status of people in isolated areas of Puerto Rico. Survey of Barrio

Mavilla, Vega Alta, Puerto Rico (with Fernández, N. A., Burgos, J. C., Plough, I. C., and Asenjo, C. F.). *Am. J. Clin. Nutr.* 17:305, 1965.

In Spanish

Deficiencias en la Dieta Tipica y Como Corregirlas (deficiencies in the typical diet and how to correct them). *La Revista de Agricultura* 41:8 (Enero–Diciembre), 1950.

Mejor Arroz, Mejor Salud (better rice, better health). San Juan, P.R.: P.R. Dept. of Instruction, 1951.

Alimentos para su Familia (foods for your family) (with others). San Juan, P.R.: P.R. Dept. of Instruction, 1952.

Cabras—Crielas para Leche (goats—raise them for milk) (with others). San Juan, P.R.: El Servicio de Extensión Agrícola, Univ. of Puerto Rico, 1954.

Leche sin Grasa (skim milk) (with others). San Juan, P.R.: P.R. Nutrition Comm., 1956.

Cuales Son las Mejores Hortilizas? (which are the best vegetables?) San Juan, P.R.: Cafe Rico, 1959.

ADDENDUM: PUBLICATIONS SINCE DR. ROBERTS'S DEATH

Energy intakes of well-nourished children and adults (with Wait B, and Blair R). *Am J Clin Nutr* 2:1383, 1969.

Nutrición, Torres RM (trans). Río Piedras, PR, Univ. of Puerto Rico, 1981.

APPENDIX 2
Lydia J. Roberts Memorial Lectures, Puerto Rico

1966	Dr. William J. Darby Nutrition Problems of International Importance, Including Some Consideration of World Food Supply and Population Approaches to the Estimation of Nutritional Requirements in the Human Being
1967	Dr. Charles Glenn King Frontiers in Nutrition—Research, Education, Action The Search for Nutrition Programs that Work
1968	Dr. E. Neige Todhunter Nutrition Education, Progress and Prospects Nutrition Education for Everyone, Methods and Media
1969	Dr. Ruth M. Leverton Dimensions of the New Protein Problem Nutrition, Learning, and Performance
1970	Dr. Arnold E. Schaefer Malnutrition: A Social, Economic, and Health Problem Nutritional Problems in Vulnerable Population Groups in the USA
1971	Dr. Ramón M. Suárez Lipids and Coronary Cardiopathies Dietary Treatment in Cardiovascular Diseases
1972	Dr. Charlotte Young Body Composition Studies of the Female The Unsolved Problems of the Obesities—Old and New Aspects
1973	Dr. Bertlyn Bosley Nutrition, Human Welfare, and Economics The Past Is Prologue—Planning and Evaluation of Nutrition Programs

1974 Agr. José Vicente-Chandler
The Potentiality of Puerto Rico for the Production of Food
Basic Problems in the Local Production of Food

1975 Dr. Jaime Benítez
Lydia Roberts and the Vocation of Service

1976 Dr. Pedro Rosso
Biochemical Aspects of Fetal and Prenatal Growth and Development
Nutrition and Mental Development

1977 Jean A. S. Ritchie
Nutrition Education in a Hungry World
Realism: The Keyword in Nutrition Education

1978 Dr. Daphne A. Roe
Drug Nutrient Interaction and Incompatibilities
Nutritional Problems in Alcoholics

1979 Dr. Nevin S. Scrimshaw
Synergism of Nutrition and Infection
Protein-Energy Relationships in Human Nutrition

1980 Dr. Mario Rubén García Palmieri
Nutritional Aspects of Coronary Disease in Puerto Rico

1981 Dr. Diva Sanjur
Patrónes de Consumo de Alimentos e Ingesta de Nutrientes en Familias Puertorriqueñas, Treinta y cinco Años Después, 1946–1981

1982 Dr. Myron Winick
Nutrition and Pregnancy
Nutrition and Brain Development

1983 Dr. Jaime Ariza Macías
Evolución de la Situación Alimentaria Nutricional de Puerto Rico. Enseñanzas Obtenidas y Perspectivas Futuras

1984 Dr. José Miguel García Castro
Posible Deficiencia de Ácido Fólico Intracelular como Etiología de los Defectos de Cierre del Tubo Neural
Defectos de Cierre del Tubo Neural y la Dieta. Situación en Puerto Rico

1985 Dr. Samuel J. Fomon
Nutrition and Growth
Iron Nutrition in Infancy

1986 Dr. James Rozovski
Influence of Nutrition on the Process of Aging
Nutrition and Aging

1987 Dr. M. C. Nesheim
The Relation of Nutrition and Parasitic Infection
Recent Developments in Nutrition Research

1988 Dr. Eduardo Santiago-Delpín
Nutrición e Inmunidad: Paradigma Actual
Como Alteran los Lípidos Dietarios el Sistema Inmunológico

1989 Dr. Evelyn Lorenzen

APPENDIX 3
Lydia J. Roberts Memorial Lectures Series, Chicago

1980 Victor Herbert, MD, JD
Nutrition Politics, the Law and Nutrition Science

1982 Norman Kretchmer, MD, PhD
Food, Nutrition, and Evolution

1983 Hamish Munro, MD, DSc
Nutrition and Aging: The Challenge

1984 Samuel J. Fomon, MD
Nutrition Requirements for Growth

1985 Doris H. Calloway, PhD
Controversy About Nutritional Needs During Pregnancy: Hcw Much Food Do Pregnant Women Require?

1986 DeWitt S. Goodman, MD
Vitamin A and Retinoids in Health and Disease

1987 James D. Cook, MD
Iron Nutrition: Too Little/Too Much

1989 Scott M. Grundy, PhD, MD
Dietary Prevention of Coronary Heart Disease: Changing Concepts

APPENDIX 4
Honors and Awards

1938 Borden Award

By direction of the American Home Economics Association

For studies with institution children demonstrating that supplemental daily feeding of one quart of milk produces considerable gains in weight and height, improved bone development and less tooth decay than does supplemental feeding of one pint daily, and that a full quart of milk daily has protective value in children's diets.

At 31st Annual Meeting of the American Home Economics Association, June 30, 1938.

1945 Citation for Public Service

Conferred by the Alumni Association of the University of Chicago

The Alumni Association of the University of Chicago holds that a university education should be the training and inspiration for future unselfish and effective service to the community, the nation and humanity; and

That men and women in accepting the privilege of a university education assume also the obligation to society to exercise leadership in those civic, social and religious activities that are essential to a democracy.

Lydia J. Roberts

an alumnus of the University of Chicago, having, in the judgment of the Alumni Association, demonstrated a practical acceptance of these obligations and responsibilities by public spirited citizenship, is hereby declared a worthy alumnus and awarded the alumni citation of

Useful Citizen

In making this citation the Alumni Association acknowledges with pride the service which has reflected credit on the University and its alumni.

Awarded by the Alumni Association of the University of Chicago on the recommendation of its College Division, June 6, 1945.

1952 Marjorie Hulsizer Copher Award
Presented by The American Dietetic Association

In recognition of a distinguished leader and teacher of human nutrition; exponent of ideals of The American Dietetic Association; pioneer in the development of nutrition work with children; and outstanding contributor to the establishment of sound national and international policies concerning nutrition. Her unusual ability to interpret scientific information to devise methods of applying the principles of nutrition to human needs has led to the improvement of human welfare. Because of her broad interests and ambitious spirit many have been inspired to follow her leadership.

Margaret A. Ohlson, President
October 24, 1952

1952 Altrusa Club of San Juan, Puerto Rico
Cited for her work in the field of Home Economics in Latin America.

1952 Lydia J. Roberts Essay Award
Named in her honor in recognition of her outstanding contributions in the field of child nutrition. The award, funded by the Gerber Products Company, was made annually by The American Dietetic Association, beginning in 1952 and continuing for twenty years. It was awarded for the best essay on the history of nutrition and dietetics.

1952 National honorary membership in Omicron Nu, Honor Society in Home Economics conferred for

a most distinguished career. . . . able administrator . . . effective teacher . . . fluent speaker . . . an eager and painstaking research worker and director.

1957 Marshall Field Award

In recognition of fundamental and imaginative contributions to the well-being of children

The Marshall Field Award

in physical and mental development is awarded to

Lydia J. Roberts

scientist and scholar, teacher and researcher, able in applying broad knowledge to specific problems, she has in the years since retirement devoted her considerable skill in improving the nutrition of the children of Puerto Rico.

January 24, 1957 — Ruth Field (Mrs. Marshall Field)

1957 Exemplary Citizen of the Commonwealth of Puerto Rico

Estado Libre Asociado de Puerto Rico
La Fortaleza
Designado a la Doctora Lydia Roberts
Ciudadana Ejemplar

Awarded by Governor Luis Muñoz Marín, February 27, 1957

1957 Honorary Life Member of Altrusa Club of San Juan

1958 Honorary degree of Doctor of Laws conferred by The Ohio State University, designating her an "internationally recognized authority in nutrition of children"

1965 Senior Citizen Hall of Fame, Chicago

Mayor's Citation awarded to

Dr. Lydia J. Roberts

in recognition of the honor conferred by having been chosen for the Senior Citizen Hall of Fame—1965. Issued at Chicago, Illinois, May 20, 1965

Harry M. Oliver, Jr., Chairman, Mayor's Committee for Senior Citizens — R. J. Daley, Mayor of Chicago

APPENDIX 5
Lydia J. Roberts, the Years of Her Life

1879	Born 30 June, Hope Township, Barry County, Michigan. Family moved to Martin, Allegan County, Michigan, when she was quite small. Family home in Martin was at 947 Allegan Street; the house still stands today.
1898	Graduated from Martin High School.
1899	Received a Limited Certificate in June from the Normal School (now Central Michigan University) in Mount Pleasant, Michigan.
1899–1908	Taught in rural schools in Michigan. Left Michigan for Montana, where she taught in the elementary schools in Great Falls and Miles City.
1909	Received Life Certificate from the Normal School, Mount Pleasant, Michigan.
1910	Returned to Montana. Taught third grade in Dillon, Montana, and was critic teacher in the Normal School there (now Western Montana College).
1915	Resigned from positions in Dillon, Montana.
	Enrolled at the University of Chicago, Department of Home Economics in the College of Education, as an undergraduate with advanced standing.
1917	Received the baccalaureate degree, University of Chicago. An honor student; member of Phi Beta Kappa.
	Appointed instructor, University of Chicago.
1918	Received the degree, Master of Science, University of Chicago. Title of thesis: "A Malnutrition Clinic as a University Problem in Applied Nutrition."
	Promoted to assistant professor, University of Chicago.

1928 Received the degree, Doctor of Philosophy, University of Chicago. Title of dissertation: "Nutrition Work With Children."
Publication of *Nutrition Work With Children* by University of Chicago Press.
Promoted to associate professor, University of Chicago.
Elected to membership in Sigma Xi.

1929 Appointed acting head of the Department of Home Economics, University of Chicago, following the resignation of Katharine Blunt.
Invited to membership in three committees of the White House Conference on Child Health and Protection.

1930 Promoted to professor, University of Chicago.
Appointed head of the Department of Home Economics, University of Chicago.

1933 Elected to membership in the American Institute of Nutrition.

1934 Became a member of the Committee on Foods (later Council on Foods and Nutrition) of the American Medical Association. Continued membership until 1948.

1935 Revised *Nutrition Work With Children.*

1938 Received the Borden Award.

1940 Became member of the original Food and Nutrition Board of the National Research Council, the National Academy of Science.
Conducted her first nutrition workshop under the auspices of the Kellogg Foundation and the University of Chicago in Allegan County, Michigan.

1941 As chairman of the Recommended Dietary Allowances (RDA) Committee of the Food and Nutrition Board, presented the proposed RDAs to the members of the American Institute of Nutrition at their annual meeting. Presented the proposed RDAs at the National Nutrition Conference for Defense, called by President Franklin Roosevelt.

1943 Visited Puerto Rico. M. L. Wilson, director of the US Extension Service and director of the National Nutrition Committee, asked her to look for nutrition problems on the island and to make recommendations for government action.
Returned to Puerto Rico in June to conduct a nutrition workshop.

1944 Retired from the University of Chicago in June.
Returned to Puerto Rico early in the year for a two-month stay to help reorganize the Department of Home Economics curriculum at the University of Puerto Rico.

Returned again to Puerto Rico in November and remained for six months, doing further work on the curriculum and developing new courses.

1945 Received Citation for Public Service, awarded by University of Chicago Alumni Association.

Invited by Jaime Benítez, chancellor of the University of Puerto Rico, to join the university faculty.

1946 Appointed professor and chairman, Department of Home Economics, University of Puerto Rico.

Received grant for the study of patterns of living in Puerto Rican families.

1948 Organized an Institute for Dietitians at the request of the Puerto Rico Dietetic Association.

1949 *Patterns of Living in Puerto Rican Families* published.

Conducted three workshops for teachers concurrently, one on nutrition, one on home improvement, and one on home food production.

1950 Repeated the three workshops for teachers held in 1949.

Conducted workshop for nutrition workers from the Caribbean area.

1951 Sent by the US State Department (along with Marjorie Heseltine of the US Children's Bureau) to Trinidad as consultant to the government regarding programs in nutrition and home economics.

Represented the United States at Conference on Nutrition Problems in Latin America, held in Caracas, Venezuela.

Honored by The American Dietetic Association with an award established by the Gerber Company, "Lydia J. Roberts Essay Award."

1952 Received Marjorie Hulsizer Copher Award, conferred by The American Dietetic Association.

Retired as head of the Department of Home Economics, University of Puerto Rico.

Served as chairman of Conference on Home Economics and Education in Nutrition, Trinidad, 30 June to 5 July, sponsored by the Food and Agriculture Organization (FAO) and the Caribbean Commission.

Accepted invitation of Inter-American Institute for Agricultural Sciences, Turrialba, Costa Rica, as consultant in home economics for Latin America.

Elected to honorary membership in Omicron Nu.

1953 Directed a three-month training course for people from the Caribbean area at the University of Puerto Rico, sponsored by FAO, the Caribbean Commission, and the University of Puerto Rico.

Designated Chairman of the US Delegation to the Third Joint Food and

Agriculture Organization/World Health Organization Latin American Nutrition Conference at Caracas, Venezuela, by the US Department of State.
Represented the United States at the Conference on Nutrition Problems in Latin America, Rio de Janeiro, Brazil.
Organized an FAO-sponsored course of study in nutrition for the University of the West Indies.

1955 Spent six weeks in Uganda, sponsored by FAO, as consultant in family living, nutrition, and women's education.

1956 Wrote the Uganda report in Rome, while a guest of Jean Ritchie.
Told Governor Luis Muñoz Marín of her desire to raise the standard of living of families living in isolated rural areas.

1957 Named Exemplary Citizen of the Commonwealth, an honor conferred by the government of Puerto Rico. Only one person had received this award previously.
Received Marshall Field Award.
Made Honorary Life Member of the Altrusa Club, San Juan.

1958 Received honorary degree, Doctor of Laws, conferred by The Ohio State University
Recognized by Governor Luis Muñoz Marín for her work in the isolated community, Doña Elena, in his address to the legislature.

1960 Appointed chairman of the newly established Commission for Improvement of Isolated Communities by Governor Luis Muñoz Marín.

1962 Completed the first five years of the Doña Elena Project.
Elected Fellow of the American Institute of Nutrition.

1963 *The Doña Elena Project* was published.

1965 Died 28 May 1965. Stricken at her desk at the University of Puerto Rico, she died a few hours later of an aortic aneurysm.
Commemorated by Chancellor Jaime Benítez in his commencement address, University of Puerto Rico.
Memorial Resolution passed by the Assembly of Delegates of the American Home Economics Association, 25 June.

1966 First Lydia J. Roberts Memorial Lecture in Puerto Rico.

1980 Lydia J. Roberts Memorial Lecture Series established by Committee on Human Nutrition and Nutritional Biology, University of Chicago, with support through a grant from the Quaker Oats Company.

INDEX